Can You Feel My Tears

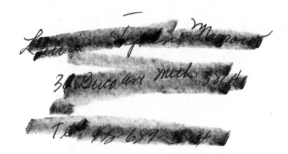

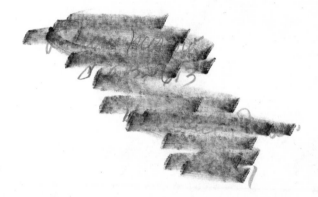

Can You Feel My Tears

My Husband's Courage And Determination To
Defy Death....and The Strength Our Love Gave
Him To Fight.

Veronica —
Always walk
in the sunshine
and let your
heart cherish each
day.
Lauri

Lauri Merrow

ISBN 1-59457-503-7
Library of Congress Control Number: 2004108108
North Charleston, S.C.
BookSurge LLC

To order additional copies, please contact us.
BookSurge, LLC
www.booksurge.com
1-866-308-6235
orders@booksurge.com

Can You Feel My Tears

With love to Danielle, Jim, Dawn and Becky...
so that you will know why mommy and daddy
were away for so long.

FOREWORD

There comes a time in everyone's life that they start to feel comfortable with the cards destiny has dealt to them. That is probably the way we felt. Sure, we had our share of everyday problems. Finances, job stress, and the day to day ups and downs that come along with being parents. It never seemed to matter though, what minor crisis was happening. We always hung in there together and rode it out. We both knew that no matter what went wrong, Steve and I would be able to see it through together.

This was the second marriage for both of us. Our previous marriages had both been, to say the least, the biggest mistakes of our lives. However, we had both been blessed with children from them and that one mistake in our lives brought us not only the children, but each other as well. Then we had two beautiful girls. Becky now two and Dawn at the fun age of five. My two children were welcomed into Steve's heart with all that he had to give, Danielle now eleven and Jimmy now at the age of nine.

Steve also has a daughter from his first marriage. Her name is Andrea. Although she had only been up to visit with him once for about a month two years prior to this, she was also a big part of his life and the love he had for her was unquestionable. She lives in Florida with her mother. Unfortunately the bitterness between Steve and his ex-wife carried over to the judgments that were made for an awful long time. Now, however, the lines of communication have been opened and the relationship between Steve and his daughter has been mended.

So here we are, parents of five children all together, married for almost five years and doing our best to hold what was so dear to us close to our hearts. We are bound and determined to always be there for each other and for our children. We are more than just husband and wife. We are the best of friends.

We were in the middle of planning a long overdue vacation for the two of us. We had not been away alone together in much too long. We had been saving for months for this. Our plan was to go to Hampton Beach for a week. We had spent our honeymoon there and had managed to get back up there twice more by ourselves. Both of us were looking forward to this time alone in order to rediscover ourselves.

However, life was dealing us nothing more than the simple trials and tribulations that everyone else in the world was going through.

My mother always told me, as her mother had always told her, "The good Lord never gives you anything that you cannot handle." She said, "Each day was a test, but nothing you could not pass.

Then one morning the telephone rang and we were faced with the biggest test the Lord had to offer us.

He paused at the door and turned to look at me. "I feel as though I'm forgetting something." With a shrug of his shoulders he said, "I love you! See you tonight."

As the door closed I got up and went to the window. Danielle and Jimmy were already in the truck waiting patiently with our friend Al. Steve would be dropping off the two kids at their father's on his way to work. The truck revved its engine once more before pulling out and taking off down the street.

I turned around to assess the amount of housework I had to tackle. With the sky as gray as it was, the two little ones would be content to stay in the house. First things first, laundry needed to be caught up and the dishwasher was full. I wanted to get things in order today so that tomorrow all I had to do was pack our suitcase. Hampton Beach was only two days away. This vacation was long overdue.

The two girls were quietly watching Saturday morning cartoons. I sorted the laundry and brought the first load of laundry to the basement to wash. As I came upstairs, I noticed the sky getting darker and a light mist was beginning. I emptied the dishwasher and got the second load of laundry together. As I was about to bring it downstairs the phone rang. I went to the living room to pick up the call.

The man's voice on the other end was unfamiliar. "Is this Laura Merrow?"

I hesitated; I was not in the mood to deal with a bill collector or a solicitor. I wanted to hang up but decided to take the call anyway. "This is Laura Merrow, who am I speaking to?"

"Mrs. Merrow, this is Mike Madden at the store." It was one of Steve's supervisors and his voice was very serious. My heart jumped to my throat. "I hate to be calling you like this, but something's happened to Steve."

My legs started to shake. I leaned against the wall for support. "Is he okay?" My voice was shaking, "What happened?"

"Please, don't panic. He's had some type of a seizure."

This was not happening. Dawn and Becky started running around at my feet. My legs felt like rubber, my mind was spinning. I picked up the phone and went in the kitchen so the girls would not see me upset.

"Mrs. Merrow?" the voice on the phone was shaking too. "I need to know if Steve's had any history of epilepsy or diabetes."

"No. Nothing like that, not at all. Is he okay? Where are my kids?"

"Kids? I haven't seen them." I could hear him asking someone if they had seen them. "No one has seen them. Were they supposed to be here?"

"Well, no. Steve was bringing them to see their father." My hands would not stop shaking. "Is Steve okay?!" I was panicking; Steve was fine when he left.

"I don't know. He complained of being dizzy. He came inside and put his head down. We went to get him a chair and his legs gave out."

Nothing was registering with me. What the hell was going on? "You're sure my kids didn't see this? Where's Al?"

The voice was getting shaky again. "Al isn't here. He is on deliveries. I have a paramedic here with me and he needs to speak to you."

A paramedic? That meant an ambulance had been called. What was wrong with Steve?

"Mrs. Merrow?"

Another strange voice. The same questions. No, there is no epilepsy or diabetes in the family. No, there are no known allergies to any medications.

"We will be transporting him to one of the local hospitals. Either Union Lynn or Melrose Wakefield."

My mind was racing. "I don't want him in Lynn. Bring him

to Melrose Wakefield. Unless his is saying he wants to go to Union Lynn."

The paramedic on the other end of the phone was scaring me. "No, he isn't really coherent."

"Please, tell me, is he okay?" My voice was really shaking now. I couldn't cry. The girls were right beside me and I didn't want them upset.

"We're not sure what caused the seizure Ma'am. We are going to get to the hospital as quickly as possible. How long will it take you to get there?"

There was no way I could drive there by myself. I would have to call Sue. "I don't know, about an hour or so."

The next few minutes seemed like hours. I called Sue first. Her mother answered the phone. Sue was in bed.

"I'm sorry Mrs. Gaumond, but could you please wake her up? It's very important." I couldn't think. I was trying to stay calm so that Dawn and Becky wouldn't pick up on what was going on. I quickly explained to Sue what was happening. She was pulling up out front ten minutes later.

The second phone call was to Linda. Linda was always there for us when we needed her. She was as good a friend as anyone could ask for. I'd put some things together for the girls and bring them over to her. She'd be able to watch them while I went to the hospital.

The phone rang. It was Linda again. She was apologizing but felt that she had to call my Mom and Dad. They would meet me at the hospital.

Dawn and Becky were quickly dropped off at Linda's. I glanced at my watch. Nine o'clock. It had only been forty-five minutes since Mr. Madden had called me. We would be at the hospital by ten o'clock.

Sue was a good friend. She kept saying that everything would be okay. By the time we pulled up at the hospital I was convinced that they were exaggerating about Steve's condition, and that he was going to be fine. It just couldn't be that bad. Steve had to be alright. What I should have realized was that the nightmare was just about to begin.

I ran up to the nurses' station in the emergency room. "My name is Laura Merrow, my husband was just brought in."

"What's your husband's name?" She turned to look at her patient register.

"Steven. Steven Merrow." My heart was racing. I felt Sue walking up behind me.

The nurse put the register down. "Mrs. Merrow, please have a seat. I'll get the doctor to come out and speak with you."

I didn't want a seat. "Where is my husband?! Is he alright?" I wanted answers. This nurse was asking me to wait for a doctor.

She leaned her head into the back room. "The wife is here!" She turned around and said, "Please, have a seat, and the doctor will be with you shortly."

As I turned to where the nurse had motioned, a man wearing a gray suit was approaching me. "Mrs. Merrow?"

Assuming it was the doctor, I started to ask about Steve's condition.

"Mrs. Merrow, I'm sorry, I am not the doctor. My name is Craig Fraser. I am Steve's boss. I came in with him on the ambulance."

At that moment a doctor introduced himself and asked me to sit down.

I was terrified. The worst possible scenario was going through my mind. No one was letting me see Steve. No one was telling me how he was doing. Now this doctor wanted me to have a seat.

He was asking me the same questions the paramedics had asked. I was shaking inside. "Doctor, please, tell me if he is okay?!!?"

"He is stable." The doctor started to explain what had been done since he arrived at the hospital, but the only thing that I heard was the word STABLE. That meant that Steve was alive, but why couldn't I see him? What was happening behind that curtain that led to the treatment room?

The doctor was going on about his findings, "CAT scan... two abnormalities...neurosurgeons...Boston...airlift..." Nothing was really sinking in. I had to see Steve.

"Doctor, can I see him?" Nothing else mattered to me at this point. I felt as though something was being kept from me.

He looked at me and for the first time since I had been there, I realized that Steve was in a lot of trouble. Composing myself, I tried to grasp what this doctor was trying to tell me.

"Mrs. Merrow, this hospital is not equipped to treat your husband properly. There is an abnormality showing up in the CAT scan. We want to airlift him to a hospital in Boston. The ones available to you are Brigham and Women's or Massachusetts General." The doctor paused and looked at me. Perhaps he was trying to determine whether or not I comprehended the graveness of the situation. He went on to ask me which hospital I wanted him transferred to.

I hated making these decisions. What would happen if I was wrong? As crazy as it sounds, I pictured Steve being told he was at Brigham and Women's Hospital. The name made me think of pregnant women. I chose Massachusetts General. I had heard it was a very good hospital, although I didn't know of anyone who had been there.

The doctor asked me to wait until the nurses were done working with him. I felt as though my world was falling apart. I was so afraid of the doctor telling me that they had lost him.

A nurse came over to me. The doctor must have sent her to check up on me. She asked me if I was okay. I didn't know. How could I be okay? My world was crashing down around me.

I asked for the use of a phone. She pointed out a phone on the wall down the corridor. Then she looked at Sue and asked her to stay with me in case I felt faint.

I tried my parents' house first. The answering machine kicked in. They must be on their way. My next call was to Steve's older sister Linda. She was eight months pregnant and I was afraid of upsetting her. She wanted to come down but I explained that Steve was being moved to Boston, but that I wasn't sure when. I asked her to call her mother for me and told her that I would call her as soon as I knew when he was going to be moved.

As I hung up the phone I could hear moaning coming from

the other side of the hall. It sounded like Steve but I couldn't be sure. Quietly, I walked over to the entrance of the treatment room. The curtain was still drawn, but not completely. All that was visible were the patients' feet.

Suddenly a voice screamed, "Get those FUCKING needles away from me!!!" It was Steve! I ran to the curtain and the nurses working on him knew that I must be his wife and let me in.

Steve was white as a ghost. His arms were thrashing at the nurses as they were trying to hook up an IV. There were three of them. One at each shoulder and the third was trying her best to find a vein to start the IV with.

I walked slowly to the bed and grabbed his hand. His hand squeezed mine and he looked at me. "Make sure the gate is closed!" he exclaimed. I didn't know what he was talking about.

"Steve, it's me. I'm here. You are gonna be okay. You have to let these ladies do what they have to do. Let them take care of you." I was only saying words. I didn't understand what was going on. All I knew was that he had to relax. His eyes met mine for the first time. There was something in his eyes I had never seen before. Something in the eyes I always looked in for my strength. They now held something new to me. Fear.

"I love you, Steve." The tears wanted to flow, but I kept blinking them back.

"I love you too, Princess." His grip loosened and he seemed to drift off to sleep.

A nurse came over to me with a chair. "Honey, sit down here. He is going to slip in and out like that for a while. He's been given Dylanten for the seizures and it makes you tired for a while."

I didn't understand. She was talking as if he had more than just the one seizure at the store. I asked her about it and she told me that he had two more at the hospital. She really didn't know what to say to me. My face must have had panic written all over it. She simply patted my shoulder and went back to her work.

I looked at Steve lying there. How could this be happening?

A nurse told me to keep talking to him and to try and reassure him that he was okay and that he was in a hospital.

I heard footsteps coming up behind me. "Laura?"

I turned around. Daddy!! Behind him was my mother! My parents were here!

"Is he all right?" my father asked. "What happened?" My father was as white as Steve was and he looked scared. Really scared.

"I don't know." I said. "It's not good. They want to bring him to Boston." I could hear my voice shaking.

My mother took me by the shoulders and guided me out to the hallway. I looked at her. She looked as though she had been crying. I couldn't do that. I was afraid to let the tears flow. I knew how much Steve hated a woman to cry. He couldn't deal with it.

I tried to explain to them the little bit that I knew. I didn't really understand why this was happening. I introduced them to Sue and Mr. Fraser.

After a few minutes my mother told me that they had called my sister Peggy to get directions to the hospital and she was going to call her and let her know what was going on. She asked if I had called my friend Linda yet, or any of Steve's family.

"Well I called his sister and she was going to call my mother-in-law," I started, "Mom I don't know what to say to anybody!" She looked at me as I tried to catch my breath. "I am so scared, if I get on the phone to them, I'll only get them panicky." My reserve had been exhausted and the tears just rolled down my face. "Mommy, what if he…"

My father came over and put his arm on my shoulder, "Shhhh…he is going to make it. Do you understand me? He has to."

My mom looked at me and could tell that I was in no condition to be making these phone calls. "Why don't you write down all the phone numbers and I will make the calls for you" she said.

I took a piece of paper and a pen out of my purse and did as she asked. My mother was being terrific. She seemed as though she was in control. I knew that I wasn't, so I let her do what she knew had to be done. She got on the phone and called everyone and caught them up on what was happening with Steve.

I walked around the corner to the treatment rooms and saw Steve's doctor looking at some type of X-ray. There were numerous views of a skull. It had to be Steve's I stood beside him trying to understand what he was saying to a nurse with him. He turned to me realizing that I was listening and tried to explain to me what he was looking at.

"These are like looking at a cross section of your husband's skull and brain," he said. "These are the films of the CT-scan."

He tried to help me understand the proportions of what I was seeing by letting me know where the nose and ears would be.

He brought my attention to a small black dot right in the center of one of the shots. "This small dot is the abnormality that is causing the problem. It's an aneurysm. The fact that it is in the center could make things extremely difficult. I am positive that it will need to be treated surgically." His voice trailed on, but I was focused on that tiny black dot which was putting my husbands' life in danger.

I turned and looked back at Steve. "Can I be with him?" I tried to explain to the doctor that they might have an easier time working on Steve if I was able to be next to him. I seemed to have a calming affect on him. The doctor shook his head. He started to say something but a commotion began then because Steve started to yell and scream. He was sitting up on the bed pulling some type of tubing device out of his throat! He heaved it across the room and then tried to yank the IV line out of his arm. It took three nurses to put him back down and restrain his hands

He kept screaming again. "No more FUCKING NEEDLES!!!!"

I turned around and ran back out to the waiting area. It had been quite obvious that everybody had heard him.

Sue came over to me, she had been crying. She told me that

someone from the admitting office had been there looking for me. "Why don't I walk over with you while they finish working on Steve?"

"Where is it," I asked.

"Come on, I'll go with you. You need to get away from this for a couple of minutes."

So the two of us went to admitting. We sat at a desk with someone punching things into a computer. She told us that she had taken his drivers license and hospital card and taken most of the information from that.

She had a few simple questions to ask and we were done. I found a soda machine and got a Coke.

When we got back to the emergency area I had to go outside and have a cigarette. Everybody followed me.

I tried to drink my soda but could not seem to swallow it. I offered it to Sue. By doing that though, set my mother into a line of questions about how I felt. She was concerned about my well-being.

Everyone tried their best to comfort me. As hard as they tried the only comfort I was finding was in the fact that they were there with me. I felt as though I had someone else to lean on. People who would help remind me that I had to hold myself together.

I wanted to get back inside though. My mother wanted me to catch my breath. I told her that I would feel better if I at least knew what they were doing to him.

I put my cigarette out and went back inside. There were more people in the waiting area and I could not bring myself to sit with them. I walked to the corner of the trauma room.

I could not see past the team of nurses and doctors that were around him. I could hear him yelling again. They must be trying to put that tube back in his mouth. I wished that I could be with him.

"Get that fucking thing away from me!!" he was screaming.

I tried to go to him, but the doctor and a nurse grabbed my arms and held me back. "Please, Mrs. Merrow let them do their job." The nurse tried to say something to calm me down but I only turned and ran outside. My parents and the others quickly followed me. I needed to calm down. My dad lit a cigarette for me. Comforting words were being said. Words of love, of friendship and of loyalty. Plans of getting me to Boston were made. Sue would be taking Mr. Fraser back to the store. She would also see Al and give him the keys to Steve's truck. Idle conversation in an attempt to soothe me.

I walked back inside and was met by a nurse. "Mrs. Merrow, there is a phone call for you. I think it is your mother-in-law." She took me to where the phone was. His mother was crying. I explained to her as much as I could. She was trying to understand, but I had to get off the phone. I had to get back to Steve. As I hung up the receiver, I simply walked past the nurses and went straight to him. I took Steve's hand. I tried to find comforting words. Tried to ease his mind while mine was so confused.

I was brought out into the hallway again, this time to sign some type of consent form for the flight to Boston. The doctor told me to try and explain to Steve about being airlifted to Boston. He felt I could make him understand.

As I turned to go back in, Steve was sitting up with a nurse beside him. He had been vomiting. The nurse was cleaning him up. He looked at me with the look of a child who had been naughty. "I'm sorry," he said. I took a cool cloth and did my best to comfort him. He lied back down.

"Steve, there is something you have to understand. They need to bring you to Boston. The headaches you have been having?" He nodded his head. "Well, there is something inside that is making you have the headaches. The doctors in Boston can take better care of you. The only thing is that they want to get you there as quickly as they can, so you will be going by helicopter."

He smiled, "Just so long as the hospital is gonna be footin' the bill for the air-fare."

I was asked again to leave the treatment room so that they could prepare him for the flight. As I was leaving the area

I passed a paramedic dressed in a flight uniform. He would be going soon.

I went back outside to where my parents and the others were waiting. I was trying so hard to accept the reality of the situation. My mother came over to me. "He will be fine. They are going to be bringing him to the best hospital around. He's a strong man who has a lot to live for. He is going to be fine." But I could tell by the look on her face that she was scared too.

"I hope so Mom," I said. I turned to Sue, "Thank you so much for getting me here, I would never have been able to do it by myself." I gave her a hug and went back inside.

As I got back into the emergency room, a stretcher was being wheeled around the corner. It was Steve. He had been wrapped in a silver insulation blanket and was harnessed to the stretcher.

I moved up beside his head, bent down and kissed him. His eyes were closed. "You hang in there! You are gonna be okay!" I don't know whom I was trying to convince, him or me. "Do you hear me? You are gonna be just fine!!"

A paramedic came over to me and handed me a map of Boston. The route to the hospital had been highlighted. I asked them before if I could go with them on the helicopter, but they had said it was going to take all four of them to transport him and that there was not enough room. I would be going with my parents. Thank God for Linda. If she hadn't called them I don't know if I would have been able to get there.

I turned back to Steve. I bent down and gave him a kiss on his lips. "I love you Steve."

His eyes fluttered open and he looked up at me. "I love you too, Princess" he said, and closed his eyes again.

They wheeled the stretcher out as I followed. My father came over to me and put his arm around my shoulders. As they put him on the ambulance I finally broke down. The tears flowed and flowed. I had no way of stopping them now. A paramedic came over and was talking to my father. I couldn't understand what he was saying, I was crying too hard. All I remember was that they would have him there in seven minutes.

My parents guided me to their car. I turned back to Sue and Mr. Fraser. I thanked them both for staying with me. They both told me the same thing. That Steve was strong and that he was a fighter. Sue gave me a hug and told me that everything would be all right.

We followed them as far as Route One and then we went in the direction the paramedic had told us to take. Straight for the Tobin Bridge.

I heard my father curse as we approached the on ramp to the Bridge. It was bumper-to-bumper and barely moving. I settled back and looked out the window. My mother turned around to me, "It shouldn't take too long," she said. I told her not to worry about it.

"Besides, Mom, it will give me a chance to calm down and get myself together before we get there."

"How can you be so calm? I would be going crazy," she said.

"I have to be calm, Mom," I said, "I'm just scared right now that he will wake up and I won't be with him."

I watched the traffic. It was basically standing still and we were still about a half a mile from the bridge. Some cars were turning off and going the wrong way down on-ramps to the bridge. I saw the look on my fathers' face as he watched them. I knew he was thinking about doing the same thing.

"Don't do it Daddy. Those people are nuts. We'll get there in plenty of time. He is in good hands."

He agreed, but he felt as though he should be something to get us there faster. It ended up taking us two hours to get through all the traffic.

With shaking hands, I smoked cigarette after cigarette. I took a deep breath and tried to pull myself together. I watched the traffic as the time passed on Steve's watch. It had been among his personal belongings. His wallet had been there too. I went through its contents. I found a ten-dollar bill and a couple of singles. I hadn't thought of money. I put the watch on and slipped the wallet into my purse.

I watched my parents exchanging looks. I assumed it was

because my father was normally uptight in traffic. It was more this time though. They were both tense and close to being panic-stricken. What I didn't know then was what the paramedic had said to my father just before we had left. If nothing else it was probably just as well because I would have lost all control.

His last words to my father were "Get her than as fast as you can, sir. As fast as you can."

Most of what happened at Mass. General's emergency room is mainly a blur. When we first arrived I rushed to the nurse's station to ask where Steve was. Just like at the other hospital, though, I was asked to please wait and that a doctor would be with me as soon as possible. We were told to have a seat. My mother took this opportunity to call my sister Peggy and my friend Linda. After about five minutes or so I went back to the nurses' station and asked if someone could please check on my husband.

"Ma'am, there are eleven beds back there and nine of them are filled. Your husband is being worked on and as soon as a doctor becomes available I will have one come out to speak with you." She apologized again for the wait and brought us to a small room off to the right of the nurses' station.

It was a small room, with a couch and an armchair. A table was in the center with an ashtray. I thought that was odd. There were no smoking signs everywhere. Why would they allow us to smoke in here? My mother commented on that as I lit a cigarette. "Mom, there would not be an ashtray in here if they didn't want us to be smoking." I knew what she meant though. It made us feel as though we were being given preferential treatment because of Steve's condition.

At that moment I heard footsteps approaching. I jumped up thinking it was a doctor or a nurse. Through the door came Steve's sisters Linda and Diane. His mother followed them. I felt their arms embracing me, asking if I had heard anything. I shook my head and filled them in with what little information I did know.

After a while, his mother got up to stretch her legs. It was warm and smoky in there. I turned to his sister Diane, who was about to graduate from nursing school, and asked her what she thought. She asked me if they were going to put a shunt in. She explained what it was and I told her I didn't know.

I could hear his mother speaking to someone at the nurses' station. I went out to where she was standing. She was asking when she would be allowed to see her son. The nurse motioned to me and told us that as soon as she got the okay from the trauma center, she would let his wife in. His mother insisted on being allowed back there to see him, "That is my son, his wife was with him already at the other hospital, I think I should be able to see him for at least a minute or two. He should know his mother is here." The nurse told her she would see what she could do.

So there we sat. After what seemed like an eternity, a doctor came in to speak to us. She looked at me, "Are you Mrs. Merrow?"

I nodded, unable to speak, afraid to hear what she was going to say.

She started by telling the family what I already knew. She explained about an abnormality called an aneurysm. It was leaking fluid into Steve's brain. That was what had caused the seizures. Most of what she said that day I couldn't remember other than the fact that they would need to surgically correct it. He would be transferred shortly up to the Neuro-surgical Intensive Care Unit.

"When can I see him?" I asked.

She said she would come out and get me when the nurses were through working on him and that it shouldn't be that much longer.

My mother asked me to call my friend Linda. She said that Linda needed to hear my voice. She came with me to the pay phone while I made the call.

I remember a woman, who said she was from admitting coming over to me while I was on the phone. I started to apologize to Linda, but I knew it was okay. I would stay on the phone with her for another minute or two. With the two of us, as long as we were in touch during a crisis and able to hear the other speak, it seemed to be enough. We shared a connection that was strong enough to endure any tragedy, as long as we were there for each other. The woman from admitting wanted to make sure that the hospital had all of the correct information for the insurance company. I told her not to apologize. At least someone was having me do something for my husband, even if it was just signing forms.

When I went back to the desk, the doctor was there to escort me and one other person, his mother, back to the trauma center. She said we could only stay for one minute.

My heart was pounding, his mother was following me but I did not notice her. All I saw was the corridor in front of me, which would finally lead me to my husband.

When we reached the trauma center the doctor stopped and told us to wait by the desk. While we waited, I looked around. The room was buzzing. Nurses and doctors were bustling from one end to the other. I watched which way the doctor went and saw her disappear behind a curtain. She came out in a moment and motioned for us to come in. My legs felt like dead weights.

When I reached the curtain I thought I was going to faint. I took a deep breath and looked at a nurse. She said it was okay to come in, but to try and not trip on any of the cords on the floor.

There were monitors everywhere and most of them were hooked up to Steve. When I reached the head of the bed I noticed a tube coming from both his nose and his mouth. I asked the nurse what they were for. She told me that it was a routine procedure in cases that involved seizures and head injuries of my husbands' magnitude. He was heavily sedated and would not be able to talk to me. She did tell me however, that as far as she knew that he could hear me.

I looked at his face. His eyes were partially open and they looked like they were glazed or had something in them. I didn't ask and I still don't know what they had done to his eyes, if anything, but I'll always remember what it looked like. I turned and looked at his mother. She saw it too. I could tell by the look on her face.

I stood by him for a moment or two then I bent down and kissed his forehead. I whispered to him how much I loved him and that I was not leaving. I told him I would be with him till he went home. I gave him one more kiss and turned around and looked for the door. I had to find the hallway. I had to get away for a minute. I got as far as the door to the trauma center and my legs just didn't want to go any further. I leaned up against the wall and cried. I didn't care who was there or who saw me, my world had just been turned upside down. The tears flowed down my cheeks. His sisters were there beside me and helped me get down the corridor. I didn't want to leave him there.

It would be at least an hour or two before they were going to get him upstairs to I.C.U. He would be going to radiology for an angiogram. This would give them a better picture of what was going on. They would be inserting a dye into his blood vessels through a catheter. The catheter was inserted into an artery, which led to the brain. The test alone would take about an hour. They gave me a consent form to sign.

Everyone thought it would be a good idea to get me out of the hospital during this test. They wanted me to eat. Food was the last thing on my mind, but I went with them. They led and I followed. I knew they were right. It was late in the afternoon and I hadn't eaten all day. Even then, I still couldn't eat I had all I could do to swallow half a bowl of soup.

I had to get back to the hospital. I had to be with Steve. His sister Linda was sitting across from me and reached into her purse. She took something out and handed it to me. "I want you to hold on to this until Steve gets better," she said, "Diane gave it to Dad when he was baptized a Catholic."

Steve's dad was Protestant, but had been baptized a Catholic just before he passed away in the hospital. I looked down at what she had handed to me. It was a silver crucifix. I closed my hand around it and thanked her.

I tried to think of what I was going to do. The doctors were talking about surgery. I knew I hadn't signed any forms as far as that were concerned. I also knew that I hadn't spoken to anyone here about his medical history. I had to get myself together. What would Steve want me to be doing? What would he do if the roles were reversed? These answers were easy. Ask questions and get answers from everyone. He was going to want to know what the hell had happened to him and he would be asking me a lot of questions. The last thing he was going to need would be a wife who fell apart during a time in his life that he needed her most.

So that is what I did. A nurse that first day suggested that I keep a notebook. As his wife, I had been appointed the spokesperson for the family. A notebook, she said, would help me keep track of not only my questions and answers, but also questions the other family members had. She also told me to write down the different procedures that Steve would be going through so that I would be able to explain them to everyone.

However, my notebook became more than that. It became my lifeline. Everything went into it right from the beginning. A small scratch pad became a larger notebook, and then there were two of them. It reads a lot like a layman's medical chart to start and then as time wore on, a journal.

Even the doctors noticed that I was putting everything down. They would help my by slowing down with their explanations and eventually helping me with the spelling of different medical terms.

Throughout this story, I share each page of my notes. Word for word and page by page, the nightmare that we began to call our life and how it touched those around us.

SATURDAY MAY 16, 1992

Aneurysm is leaking fluid – causing pressure
Aneurysm is off main vessel to brain
(bulging more than a common aneurysm would – looks like
three aneurysms the way it is bulging.)
He will need surgery.
"drain" to relieve pressure – VENTRICULOSTOMY

I went back to my mothers' house that night. I can't say that I remember much of what happened other than the fact that arrangements were made for me to stay there while Linda, my good friend, took care of my children.

They couldn't operate on Steve that night because he was not stable enough. They found out late in the day that he was a smoker, which meant that his lungs need to be cleaned out.

I thought about the events of the day. I remembered when a Doctor Shummaker came out to the waiting area to talk to us...

A nurse accompanied him, and they had been in radiology during the angiogram on Steve.

"Mrs. Merrow?" He asked us to step into the corridor so that he could speak to us alone. He explained where the leak was coming from. The entire family stood around me. Every word the doctor spoke pierced my heart like a knife. Steve was in a lot of danger. He had a machine helping him to breathe and a bubble in his brain that was leaking. His mother kept stopping the doctor to ask questions. She basically wanted this doctor to tell us that everything was going to be okay and that Steve would be fine.

Finally, between my questions and the doctors' explanations, the doctor stopped and looked at my mother-in-law and then back at me.

"Listen," he said. His face was stone cold. "Your husband is a very sick man. This is a very serious condition he has. You have to realize one thing right now and that is that he may die."

At that point, my legs buckled, and the room went around. I reached out for Steve's sister, Diane. "Oh, my God, no." This doctor had finally said the one thing that no one had dared to say all day long.

I vaguely remember someone getting me a chair. A nurse was patting my hand while the doctor knelt in front of me. He was being very nice but kept an extremely serious tone with me. He was letting me know exactly what they had seen. He was sorry for his bluntness but felt that he had to make sure we understood.

He handed me a consent form to sign. I would allow them to perform what was called a ventriculostomy. He explained the procedure and all of the risks.

"The ventriculostomy is a surgical procedure which is done right at his bedside in I.C.U. A small incision will be made on the top of his head and small hole drilled through the skull. Then we will place a catheter tube into the area where the fluid is building up. The fluid, cerebral spinal fluid, will then drain into a bag." He looked at me to make sure I was listening, and that I understood. He went on to tell me that Steve was hooked up to a ventilator. A machine was helping him to breathe. That was the reason for the tube that I had seen in the emergency room. He also had a tube going into his mouth and down to his stomach. It was draining anything from his stomach to prevent him from vomiting again.

I looked down at the consent form when the doctor was finished with his explanations. I took the pen from his hand

and put my name where he indicated. At that point all I could think of was "anything, dear Lord, anything, just keep my Steve alive."

SUNDAY MAY 17, 1992

Sat with a Doctor Ogilvy. He explained surgery –
Either through the side of the head or through the nose (a
new procedure which was developed at Mass. General)
Surgery – transfacial clipping at the base of the aneurysm
Could develop a VASO – SPASM up to at least one week
after surgery

Vaso-spasm was explained to me this way: the fluid, which is
leaking from the aneurysm, sits against the blood vessel. For
some reason, which doctors have not come to understand yet,
the vessel will contract when blood passes through it instead
of expanding properly. If this were to happen, it would cause a
stroke.

If the drain (ventriculostomy) does not work properly –
Hydrocephalus would develop. Fluid would build up in the
areas of the brain called ventricles and would cause the brain
to swell.
If this happened, then a shunt would have to be put in.
A shunt was a permanent drainage tube. Surgically put in,
Would perform the same thing as the ventriculostomy.
*(it was not definite at this time that this would be
necessary)
He would need a tracheal tube put in for the surgery. Only
temporarily.

Seven doctors would be performing the surgery.
A plastic surgeon, and Ear/Nose/Throat specialist (for the
sinuses)
Three neurosurgeons and the anesthesiologists
Plus the nursing team
Sunday night:
Response good
Stable
Ventricles smaller – this was a good sign
Aspiration pneumonia in the right lung only

Aspiration pneumonia occurs when a patient breathes in their own vomit. It would get into the lungs, thereby causing the pneumonia. The nurse who explained this to me could not understand how he could contract this because there was no record of him vomiting. I explained to her the incident at Melrose/Wakefield Hospital yesterday. She informed the doctor.

The upper portion of the right lung had collapsed.
On the respirator – this would help correct this
Chest s-ray on lungs showed improvement
Lungs unable to tolerate surgery until Tuesday.
On a drug called Barbarchurate which would lower his
blood pressure
Have to suction his lungs every one to two hours. Blood
pressure has to be low because of the leak, suctioning of course
causes his blood pressure to rise.

I met Doctor Ogilvy this morning. I was very hesitant to accept him as Steve's doctor. H appeared to be about thirty five but not much over forty. I was to find out later on that he is the best neuro-surgeon around. Steve could not have been in better hands.

Dr. Ogilvy met my dad and me outside of the I.C.U. doors and looked around for a private spot to discuss things with us.

He guided me down some corridors saying that he knew of a nice quiet place that would be more comfortable and there would be less of a chance of being interrupted.

He was extremely patient with me. His explanations of what was happening to my husband were clear and to the point. He didn't try to treat me like the "poor wife". I think he knew better. I sat there with my pen and paper writing down as much as I could. He made a diagram of what a common aneurysm would look like. He told me that Steve's didn't look like that. His was bulging and took on the appearance of a cluster of aneurysms.

He knew I was scared. He told me that each procedure would be explained to me in detail as they happened. I told him that I wanted to be informed every step of the way. That it was extremely important for me to be able to explain things to Steve when this was all over.

He told me that there were two different ways of approaching the aneurysm. One would be the most commonly practiced. That would be when they went through the side of the skull. In Steve's case this would be very dangerous and extremely risky. In all probability, from what I was hearing, if it was done this way, they would not be able to get to it in time.

The other, although it had been done differently before, was a new procedure developed at Mass. General. It had only been performed on three patients before this. The approach would be through the nose, then through the sinuses to the brain. Prior to this, the approach had been through the mouth. However it sounded as if this new approach was easier and made more sense.

He explained that one part of the procedure was still in the experimental stages and hadn't been perfected. It would not however, interfere with them getting to the aneurysm.

He went on to explain that after they performed what was called an M.R.I, the team would all sit down and discuss which way would be the safest way to approach the surgery. They would not perform the M.R.I., however, until they felt that Steve was stable enough for the surgery.

Monday May 18, 1992

I went crazy that day. I knew in my heart that the only way to save my husbands life was for them to operate. No one was telling me when they were going to do that. I asked a nurse if she knew when the surgery was scheduled. She only shook her head.

I went into Steve's room. My heart was breaking. He would just lie there helpless. Machines were breathing for him. I watched the monitors as they counted his heartbeats and his brain waves. It was as if it was not real. This was happening to someone else, not to me, not to us, not to my husband.

I held onto his hand and tried to talk to him. But he was motionless. He was being kept so drugged up in order to keep his blood pressure low that I wasn't even sure if he knew I was with him.

I was losing control. What were these people doing?? Why couldn't they just get things over with? My head was spinning. Steve was in so much danger! He might die!

I went back to the nurses' station and grabbed one of the nurses. "Listen to me! Someone has to know something!"

She told me to please keep my voice down. "Mrs. Merrow, what seems to be the problem?" she asked.

She told me that she was not Steve's nurse and was not sure of what was going on with his case. I stood there while she found Steve's nurse.

The same nurse came back to me and told me to wait in the corridor and that Steve's nurse would be out shortly to see me.

When I went into the corridor, Steve's friend Al was

waiting for me. I must have looked crazed "What happened?" he asked.

"They don't know what the hell they are doing in there! He has to be operated on and no one is doing it!" I was crying again.

At that moment another nurse came through the doors and said she was Steve's nurse. "Didn't the doctor explain to you that your husband was not stable enough to operate on yet?" she asked.

I couldn't believe this was happening. All I wanted was for somebody to tell me when he would be stable enough to go ahead with everything.

"Look, that is my husband in there!" I was yelling at her. "He could die! All I want is for someone to do something! I want to talk to his doctor. I want to talk to the doctor and if he can't talk to me then get someone down here who can help my husband!"

She told me to calm down. She made a telephone call and spoke to someone. Then she asked me to please have a seat in the waiting room. The doctor was unavailable but his nursing coordinator would be up in a few minutes to talk to me. Her name was Deidra Buckley.

Al was with me and told me to calm down. I guess at that point he was afraid I might punch the nurse in the face. I think I probably would have had he not calmed me down.

Pretty soon a woman with blond hair and wearing a white jacket sat down next to me. She introduced herself as Dede Buckley. Through a lot of tears and sobbing I told her that I could not understand why they had not scheduled Steve's surgery.

She just shook her head and said the one thing I had been so desperately waiting to hear, "He is scheduled for surgery at about eight o'clock tomorrow morning."

That was all that I wanted to hear. The floodgates opened again. I was sobbing uncontrollably. There was nothing that either Al or Ms. Buckley could say or do to stop them.

Dede Buckley walked me into Steve's room and then

slowly and quietly left us alone. I held his hand and looked at him lying so motionless. "Steve," I squeezed his hand, but got no response. "They will be operating on it in the morning." I told him that I was going to be seeing Doctor Ogilvy that night and that he would be going over everything with me. "Don't worry. I won't let them do anything to you that you wouldn't want. But they have to operate." The tears just rolled down my cheeks and fell onto his hand. "I can't lose you. You have to fight for me. You have to fight for us."

That night my parents were with me for the consultation with the doctor. This man would have my husbands' life in his hands tomorrow and I was not quite sure of what to say or what to ask, other than what I did.

He met us at about seven o'clock and brought us into a conference room. My parents sat down and I sat next to them. The doctor pulled a chair over and sat directly in front of me. "Finally Mrs. Merrow, he is now stable enough to withstand us going in," he started. "Let me explain what will happen."

He didn't hedge. He didn't pull any punches. I held on to every word that he said. "After seeing the films from the MRI and the angiogram we, the team and I, have decided that the best approach will be the new one. We will be going through the nose." He paused and looked at me, "That is if that's all right with you. Yours is the final decision."

I couldn't believe this man was asking me this. "Doctor, you do whatever you have to do to keep him alive."

He went on to try and explain how they would be doing the surgery. An incision would be made along the right side of the nose and under the nostrils. The nose would then be moved aside and the sinus area would be next. A specialist from Massachusetts Eye and Ear Infirmary would work on the sinuses. He would carefully move the sinuses out of the way. A bone would be broken which is located behind the sinuses. The next step would be to cut through the dura (a membrane which covers the brain).

After all of this was completed, they would be able to get to the aneurysm and clip it. The aneurysm could not be cut. If it were cut, there would be a risk of the clip slipping off. After it was clipped they would puncture the aneurysm to prevent it from filling back up again.

He went very slowly in his explanation and stopped a number of times to answer my questions and to allow me to jot down a couple of notes.

He gave me the names of all the surgeons involved and their specialties. He even took the time to make sure that I had the correct spelling.

He also explained to me that when they successfully had the aneurysm clipped they would begin the closing procedure, which was basically doing everything in reverse. This alone would take about four to five hours. The entire procedure, he said, would take anywhere from ten to twelve hours.

When he was finished he looked at me and said, "Now I have this piece of paper that I am required to have you sign. It is a terrible thing, and I don't enjoy asking anyone to sign it. It simply has a statement which says that you understand the procedure that we will be doing and it has a listing of all the risks."

He handed me the consent form. I read every word on it. Then I looked at the hand written list of risks. There were four of them noted.

Coma

Stroke

Paralysis

Hemorrhage

Next to the word hemorrhage was a small notation in parenthesis. It simply stated one thing.

Hemorrhage (death)

I looked at the doctor and pointed to his notation. "What are his chances?" I asked.

He hesitated and then said, "Well, if he gets through the surgery, he has a ninety-five percent chance of a complete recovery."

"That is not what I meant," I said. "What are his chances

tomorrow? Exactly how prepared should I be to come here tomorrow and lose my husband?"

My mother gasped. Her face went white as a sheet. "Laura, how could you ask him that?" she yelled. My father simply took hold of my hand and squeezed it tight.

I looked at my mother and said "Mom, I need to know if Steve might die." I turned my attention back to the doctor. "How prepared for that should I be tomorrow?"

The doctor turned to my mother. "You shouldn't be upset. She has asked all the right questions. She has asked more questions than most people in her position would ever consider asking." Then he turned to me and said, "I can't lie to you, this operation is very serious and very risky. Yes you should be prepared. You should also remember this. We are going to be doing our best to get him through it."

The doctor handed me his pen and I signed his consent form. "Thank you for telling me. I had to know." I handed him the form and said to him, "I realize all of the risks that are involved. I can deal with any risk on that list but one. Please, just please, keep him alive for me."

He shook my hand and asked if I had any more questions. If not then the anesthesiologist would be in to talk to me in a moment. I can remember as he was leaving, he stopped at the door and turned back to me.

"Promise me that you will hang in there." He said. "Try and get some sleep tonight, I'll try and do the same."

I smiled and told him it was a deal.

When the anesthesiologist came in, he also had a consent form for me to sign. He started to tell me what his job would be the next morning. I stopped him in mid sentence. "Listen, there couldn't be anything you are going to tell me that will top what Dr. Ogilvy just told me. Just do me one thing tomorrow."

"What's that Mrs. Merrow?" he asked.

"Keep him stable and breathing so that they can operate." With that comment, I took his pen and signed the consent form. I stood up, shook his hand and left the room.

I stopped into Steve's room before my parents brought me

back to their house for the night. I held on to his hand and told him once more how much I loved him. The tears just flowed and flowed. I kissed him, said goodnight and went out to the nurses' station. I arranged for a priest to stop by during the night to say a prayer with him. The nurse said she would take care of it. She told me to call her anytime during the night. She knew how hard this was for me and said it didn't matter why I needed to call, even if I simply could not sleep. She would be there not only for Steve, but for me as well. I asked her also if I could be allowed in to see him before the surgery started. She told me no problem.

I went back into his room. A nurse was with him. I asked her if they would be taking his ring off for the surgery. She said that they had tried to, but it hadn't come off. They were considering cutting it off. The medications had caused his hands to swell and they were afraid that the ring would cut into his finger.

I had her get some Vaseline. I covered his finger with it and with a little bit of effort, the ring slipped off. That night I found Steve's chain that held his small gold cross. I slipped both the silver cross his sister had given me, and his wedding ring onto the chain and put the chain around my neck.

At my parents' house that night, I decided to call Steve's ex-wife, Robin, and let her know what was happening. I felt as though his daughter Andrea should be prepared for what was happening to her father the next day. With each sentence I told her, I could hear her getting more and more upset. When I was through, I promised her that someone would get in touch with her when it was over. I didn't know what she should say to Andre, her daughter, but that it was probably for the best if Andrea was told something. She took my mother's phone number and asked that I send Steve her best.

My two older sisters, Peggy and Debbi, stopped by that night to see how I was holding up. They were going to be with me in the morning and would bring me to the hospital. Steve's friend Al was there with us too. We all sat around talking until I felt I could go to bed.

My sisters left with the promise of being back early to get me. Al stayed on my parents couch for the night. He would be bringing my mother to the hospital tomorrow. Somehow later that night, I fell asleep as I held on to Steve's ring.

I remember waking up in the middle of the night to find my father sitting at the kitchen table. "You can't sleep either," I said. "He has to be okay, Daddy, he just has to be. I won't settle for anything less."

But I was scared. More than scare, I was terrified. I called the hospital. Steve was stable and sleeping. They had told me in the early part of yesterday's whirlwind of explanations, that they had induced him into a comatose state. Meaning that they had drugged him so much that it gave the impression that he was in a coma. The nurse on the phone told me to try and get some sleep. That was so easy for them to say. Steve wasn't their husband.

My father went back to bed. I sat there. Alone. Suddenly a thought went through my mind. Steve and I had a conversation a few years ago about death. We talked about what we wanted the other to do if something ever happened to the other. We had talked about whether we wanted to be buried or if we wanted to be cremated.

I couldn't remember what he wanted. The conversation had been right after his father had died. I knew that it was an awful and morbid thing to have going through my mind, but I couldn't remember what he had said.

I was awake the rest of the night trying to remember...

Tuesday May 19, 1992

The morning finally came and with it came what looked like disaster. I called the nurses station to see how Steve had done during the night. The nurse covering Steve's case told me that she was just about to call me. That nothing was wrong, and for me not to panic, but that she had put a call in to Steve's doctor because his temperature was up a little.

This couldn't be happening. She told me to call back in about a half an hour or so and she would let me know if it was going to delay the surgery or not.

As I was hanging up the phone my father was coming into the room. "What happened?" he asked.

"I'm not sure. Steve's running a low temp. The nurse told me to call her back." I started to pace. "Daddy, it might delay the surgery."

My father looked at the clock. It was six thirty and he was planning on spending some time at the shop. I told him to go to work and that I would call him as soon as I knew anything.

I called the nurse back at the stroke of seven o'clock. She said that the doctor wanted to go ahead with the surgery. Steve's temperature was low grade, ninety-nine point six, and waiting would be more risky than trying to lower the temperature.

When my sisters showed up, we headed straight out to the hospital. It only took Debbi fifteen minutes to get us there.

Surgery is a go!!
Consultation with Dr. Ogilvy at seven o'clock last night
He will be going through the nose.
Risks: coma

Stroke
Paralysis
Hemorrhage – death
Will be doing a skin graft on the leg and taking some fat tissue from his hip

Test performed so far:
CT-scan (fancy x-ray)
Angiogram – will show good picture of what is going on
MRI – Magnetic Residual Imagery (3D picture of aneurysm)
Doctors involved in surgery:
Dr's Ogilvy, Barker and Crowel – neuro surgeons
Dr Joseph –Mass Eye and Ear for sinus area
Dr. Cheney – plastic surgeon
Dr. Honkenan – anesthesiologist

I had asked Daddy if I could request that the surgeons who had developed this new surgery could be called to now perform it on Steve. When I asked the nurses about it, however, I was told that the doctor who developed and perfected it was Dr. Ogilvy.

When I got upstairs, I stopped at the nurse's station to see if the priest had come in during the night. They didn't know but would call to have him come up then. When he arrived he told me that he had been there the night before but would stay with me and the two of us could pray together. Which is what we did. I prayed, I cried and he held on to my hand as we asked God to stay with Steve today and to guide the surgeons' hands.

The nurse came in to tell me it was time. I kissed Steve one more time, and turned around to leave the room.

My sisters went downstairs to the first floor with me. We found the "Gray Lobby Waiting Area" for families who were waiting for someone who was in surgery. The "room" was simply a section of the lobby partitioned off, with chairs and sofas set up for approximately thirty or so people. An older woman wearing a pink jacket sat at a small desk. She took my name and jotted it down on a clipboard next to Steve's name. She had a patient register. She was pleasant as she showed me where the coffee bar was and noted that the pastries were fresh.

My sisters and I went outside and had a cup of coffee. They tried their best to get me to eat something. I couldn't. They were hungry though, so I had my coffee while they ate.

We had grown apart over the years and had not been that close for a long time. But the love and caring that they showed me that day, I will always hold dear to my heart. Everyone that day, with all the worries that they had to deal with, held very close to me. Each one of them took turns either holding on to me or trying in their own special way to comfort me.

At about nine o'clock that morning the woman in the pink jacket came over to me to let me know that I had a phone call. It was my father. He wanted to know if the surgery was still on or not. I had forgotten to call him. I could hear him start to cry when I told him that the surgery had started about a half an hour ago. He said that he would be there as soon as he could.

At some point during the day, my mother and I took a walk. She told me a story about a man who turned gray overnight. It seems that this gentleman was about thirty years old. He had been told one day, and it was all in the same day, some very disturbing things. He was told that he lost his job, his wife was leaving him, his mother ran off with his father's best friend and his doctor told him that he only had three months left to live. The next morning he looked in the mirror and his hair had turned completely white. The shock of seeing this gave the man a heart attack and he died.

What my mother was trying to tell me was that I should keep the faith and that there would be other things to worry about tomorrow. She took my face in her hands and looked at my hair. "See, " she said softly, "No gray hair! You are going to be just fine."

She put her arm around me and we walked back to the waiting area together. Mothers are great. Always there when you need them, even when you don't think you do.

I sat down next to my sister Debbi. "You okay?" she asked. "Sure, I'm just fine."

"Look, I was going to wait and bring this out later, but maybe you need it now." She bent over and reached into her tote bag. She had loaded it up with goodies she said.

"I don't feel like looking at a magazine, Deb, but thanks." How could I possibly be able to concentrate on reading right now? "Maybe later."

"No, it's not a magazine. I found this book last night and thought it would be perfect for you to pass some time with." She smiled and kept fishing through her tote bag. She pulled out a couple of magazines a novel, some candy and then, "Here it is. The perfect book for every wife who has to wait while her husband is being operated on. When you're finished with it, give it to Steve to read." She smiled and pulled out a book and held it up. "Curious George Goes to the Hospital!"

I couldn't help but laugh and give her a big hug. Leave it to Debbi to be sure and have something to ease the tension.

Surgery began between eight thirty and nine o'clock Dede Buckley kept us informed of what was happening every two to three hours during the day.

At 7:45 am the nurses let me in to be with Steve prior to the surgery. I had a priest pray with me. Deb and Peg went to the hospital with me. Mom showed up at about ten o'clock with Al.

Kathy and Diane were there shortly after. Daddy came in at about three or four o'clock. Peg's husband Billy was there by nine that night.

I was so prepared each time I saw Dede to hear the worst. Nobody spoke about it.

I had asked Dr. Ogilvy what Steve's chances were. He said they were good if he made it through the surgery. But when I asked him if I should be prepared for the worst, he told me that I should prepare myself for anything, including the worst.

I will never want to feel the emotions of this day again. The surgery took fifteen and a half hours.
Everybody there watched me, and the clock. It is something I will never forget. When it was over, I sent everyone home. Al stayed with me to give me a lift back to Mom and Dad's.

I can remember Dede coming down to us off and on to let us know what was happening. Each time I would ask her the same thing, "Is the aneurysm clipped yet?" It was taking so long. It took hours for her to tell me that they had gotten as far as the dura, the covering to the brain.

She always came right over to me. She wanted so badly to be able to tell me what I wanted to hear. She was my personal "Florence Nightingale".

Finally, late in the day, I saw her coming around the corner, she was smiling. I got up and ran to her. She took me by the shoulders and said, "It is clipped!"

A roar of cheering and joy erupted from behind me. I turned to the family and said, "They got it!" My legs were about to give out from under me and I leaned against Dede for support. She turned me back around to face her, "It looked clean. It looked like it went very clean."

I looked at her with tears streaming down my face and asked her what she meant. She told me that it looked as though they got to it without hitting anything along the way.

She sat down with the family and me and tried to explain what she found out. It seemed that when they got to the aneurysm, it was as though there were four aneurysms instead of just one. That was how bad that damn thing looked. As she went on to explain the different happenings the only thing I can remember her saying is that this procedure would be written up in the medical books.

She explained that one of the reasons that it took so long was that once every hour on the hour they had to place the nose back where it belonged to assure proper circulation.

She also wanted us to realize that the surgery was far from over. They had put temporary clips on the adjoining blood vessels. These clips still had to be removed and they would have to watch the flow of blood to be sure that the permanent clips were tight. Then the closing procedure would begin. That would take about four to five more hours.

It seemed as though it was enough news for us to celebrate. We all hugged each other through tears of joy; we all felt the same thing. If the aneurysm had been clipped, then the worst was over.

Phone calls were made to those who were waiting at home. Steve had gotten through the worst of it, not only that but he had made the medical books.

Dede was leaving for the day but told us that when Doctor Ogilvy was through with his portion of the operation, he was going to try to come up to talk to us. It was seven o'clock.

The hours ticked away. Eight o'clock, nine o'clock. Why hadn't anyone called us? Slowly the waiting room cleared out and was left with only our family and one gentleman who was waiting for news about his wife.

No phone call. No appearance from the doctor. The longer the wait, the worse it got.

Perhaps we had celebrated too soon. Had something gone wrong after Dede left? Doctor Ogilvy's part of the operation was over with hours ago as far as I could tell. Why then wasn't he coming out to talk to us? I started to think the worst. Perhaps when they took the temporary clips off, something had happened.

My eyes stuck fast to the clock and the corridor. I tried to call the I.C.U upstairs; they didn't know anything other than that the doctor and Steve were still in the operating room.

Everyone tried to come up with a different reason for the wait. However, the longer we waited, the less people talked. We just sat and waited. I could feel everyone watching me. I would try to get up and take a walk but they didn't want to leave me by myself. I felt as though they wanted me to reassure them that everything would be okay. I couldn't do that. I felt that there was something that had gone wrong.

I went outside for a cigarette with Al. I told him of what

kept me awake the night before. He tried his best to comfort me. Nothing worked Nothing seemed to help. Debbi appeared at the door, "Laura! The Doctor is on the phone!!" She held the door as I took the stairs two at a time and bolted to the desk where the phone was. My father was holding the receiver.

"Mrs. Merrow?" the voice on the line asked.

"Yes Doctor, this is Mrs. Merrow, is Steve okay?" I could barely breathe.

"Mrs. Merrow, this is Doctor Ogilvy. The surgery is over. Your husband is still in the O.R. being prepared to be taken up to I.C.U. He should be there in about ten minutes or so."

"Doctor, is he okay, did the surgery go well?" I didn't know what to ask him. I only wanted to know if Steve was okay and if the operation was a success. He told me Steve was all right and the surgery went well.

I told him that it just didn't seem to be enough to simply say thank you.

Steve was brought back to his room.
They will let me see him in about a half hour.

It was just after midnight, so when the relief and tears had subsided, I sent everyone home. Al stayed with me. We went upstairs to the waiting room outside of I.C.U. There was a family sitting there as well. Two gentlemen with flight bags, and an older woman. The two men had just flown in, one from Atlanta. He was the oldest. Their father was in critical condition. He asked me if one of my parents was in I.C.U.

I shook my head and told him my husband had just finished being operated on.

He asked me if he had a beard. I nodded. "They wheeled him by just before you came in." At that moment a nurse came out to get me.

I wasn't sure what to expect when I walked into his room. I had visions of his head being wrapped in bandages. When I got to the door of his room, I stopped. I remember the nurse coming over to me and guiding me to the bedside. Her arm was around me as though she were afraid I would faint.

His head was not wrapped as I had expected it to be. All that was there was a bandage on the ventriculostomy. There was a splint and a bandage on his nose. They had put a tracheal tube in his throat and I could hear the ventilator pumping his breath for him.

His right eye was swollen shut and his upper lip was swollen to four or five times its normal size. The tip of his tongue was swollen and protruding out of his mouth.

My legs started to buckle and I could feel the nurses' grip tighten around my waist. I reached my hand out and touched his leg. My heart jumped!! "He moved his leg!!" I exclaimed. The nurse told me to be careful because of the graft on his upper thigh. I lifted the sheet to look at it. Maybe that was why his leg moved. It didn't matter. It moved!

Then I put my hand in his. I expected to feel the emptiness I had felt that morning because he wouldn't be able to hold my hand. I started to cry and the tears ran down my cheeks onto his arm. I am not sure if he heard me crying or felt the warmth of the tears on his arm, but at that moment his hand tried to close around mine.

"Oh my God!" I cried, "Steve? Steve, I love you! You are going to be okay!" I bent over his bed and kissed his chin. That's when I realized that they hadn't shaved his face. Dr. Ogilvy had said he would try not to but I never thought they would be able to save the beard. "Good-night sweetheart!" I thanked the nurse for letting me in to see him, turned around and left his room.

I ran out of I.C.U. ecstatic. Al was waiting for me. The tears were rolling down my face. "He's okay! He moved!" I must have sounded hysterical. "Let's go home. I have to let them know! I have to call everyone!"

Al took me back to my parents' house. They were sitting at the table waiting for me. All it took was one look at my face and they knew that Steve had gotten through okay. When they had left the hospital, as did everyone else, they thought that something had gone wrong. It had taken so long. But they knew that by my smiling face that Steve was okay.

I called his mother's house and had her get Steve's little sister out of bed. I told them both that he was still in critical condition, but that the surgery went well, and that he had moved when I touched his leg. That meant that he was not paralyzed and that he was probably not comatose. No. The doctor had not come up to see me. No. He was not out of danger yet. But yes. He was alive and he was showing initial response.

My mother had saved all the messages that had come in on the answering machine that day. There were two from Steve's ex-wife asking that we please call so that she could send her little girl to school the next day knowing how her daddy was. My good friend Midge had called asking us to let her know the outcome and that she would be praying for Steve all day. All of the messages were like that. I was in my glory. All of these people could be told one thing.

Steve was alive.

Wednesday May 20, 1992

After about three hours of sleep, Al dropped me off at the main entrance of the hospital. I was functioning on pure adrenalin. The nurses the night before had arranged for me to get in to see him early just this once. Visiting hours were normally eleven in the morning until eleven at night. Five minutes, once an hour. Immediate family only. However, where Steve had been through such a long surgery, they thought it would be okay for me to get in early this once.

I buzzed the nurse's desk from an intercom just outside the entrance to the unit. A nurse said she would be out to get me shortly. She was working with my husband.

I sat in the waiting room for what seemed like an eternity. The family from the night before were still sitting there. The flight bags were still with them as well. They must have spent the night waiting. I came to find out that the father was comatose and there was very little hope. The family would be gathering during the day. It seems that he had a living will and the oldest son was the executor. He had such a heavy burden on his shoulders, yet still took the time to talk with me about Steve. He wished me well and the best for Steve.

Finally a nurse came out and walked with me into Steve's room. I went to the side of his bed and held on to his hand. He was still under the influence of the drugs they used to put him in an induced comatose state and would probably not wake up for a few more days. They weren't giving him any pain medication because of this, basically he didn't need it until the medication had worked itself out of his system. The nurse assured me that he was not in any type of pain.

I looked around the room. There was a lot of equipment. A lot of monitors hooked up to Steve. I had the nurse explain them all to me. I wanted to be able to understand. When she started to tell me that things were routine or used words that I didn't understand, I told her that I wanted her to explain everything to me so that when Steve woke up I could explain them to him. I also told her that anything I didn't understand, I was looking up in a medical book at my parent's house. She told me everything I needed to know. How to read the monitors, what the alarms meant and at what rate they were set to go off at.

The nurse would call out his name in an effort to rouse him, but other than an attempt to open his left eye, there was no movement. He just lay there. He was so still.

It was so hard to look at him lying so still and helpless. There was no movement, no response to my touch. The hell he had to endure yesterday was just so unimaginable. I knew that even though he couldn't speak to me, he was able to hear my voice. It seemed so senseless to tell him that everything was okay. That everything was going to be all right. I had to let him know that I was there and that I loved him. Then it hit me. I sang to him. I had just finished a new song that I wrote for him. He had only heard it once or twice, but I had to try.

As I softly sang to him, I held his hand. I sang the same words over and over again...

"...I can look into your eyes, and without saying a word, know that deep within your heart, my feelings can be heard
'Cause it doesn't take a sound, to light the flame within and even though the words aren't said, the feelings still remain...."

Suddenly, without a warning, the hand I was holding began to tighten around mine. He heard me. When I stopped singing the grip got tighter as though he wanted me to continue. So I did. I sang until I couldn't sing anymore. I couldn't go on much longer, the lump in my throat was tightening. I needed to get some air. When I tried to pull my hand back, I could feel him trying to hold on. I assured him I was only going for a walk. That I would be right back.

I sang that song to him every morning he was still unconscious. Each morning we held on to each other's hands. He may have been in a comatose state, but I knew he could hear me. He always knew I was with him.

This was the beginning of our battle together. I knew that if we could hold on together, we would beat it. We had to. Our lives together had just begun. As long as I had an ounce of fight, an ounce of strength, I would continue to fight for the things that meant so much to both of us. Our love. Our children. Our future.

Lips and tongue very swollen.
Bleeding from incision on nose (expected)
Fever up to 104 degrees
Dropped to 102 degrees
On a cooling blanket
Medications: Tylenol
Antibiotics (two types)
Barbichurate
Dylanten
Inner Cranial Pressure fluctuating between 0 and 11
Drain at 11
Coughing
Breathing above respirator
Tries to open left eye.
Responds to the sound of my voice!
Questions to ask:
What caused the fever?   ***THEY DON'T KNOW***
How is pneumonia?   ***SOME***
        IMPROVEMENT
Explain if and how he will be weaned off the drain.
NOT FOR AT LEAST A WEEK
When will they be doing the next angiogram?
FRIDAY OR MONDAY

How long before he is out of danger?   **NEXT WEEK**
When will they be doing neurological exam?   **ONE IS DONE EVERY DAY BY THE NURSES AND A NEUROLOGIST EXAMINES HIM EVERY THREE DAYS**
When is the Inner Cranial Pressures expected to be at 0 and steady?   **IT SHOULD NEVER BE AT ZERO BECAUSE A NORMAL PRESSURE IS 10.**
They have done a bronchostomey – because of the fever.
This will help to clean out his lungs.
His arms and legs are moving and bending on their own.
He is having a vaso-spasm. (puts him at a high risk for a stroke)

I had set up a designated donor program for Steve. This would enable people to donate blood for him in the event that he needed any transfusions. One of the guys he works with came in to donate. His sisters couldn't and his mother was not the same blood type. I wished that I could donate.

His mother and sisters came in to see him. When Linda walked into the waiting room she handed me a yellow carnation. "I thought you could use some cheering up," she said. I went in with them to see Steve, one at a time. It was so hard. Just to be there with him, though, was helping. Something had to help him through these next few days.

While they were talking to Steve, I would watch the monitors trying to understand them more. I could remember watching his heart rate before and it had been at about 100 to 110. I thought it was odd that it was going up to about 120 or 125.

When I went out to the corridor, I asked his sister Diane what a normal heart rate was and she told me that it was about 85 to 90 depending on the person. I didn't understand. Why was Steve's up so high?

When I went back inside with his sister Linda, I stopped and asked his nurse what she thought. She explained that now that the surgery was over they were giving him medication keep his blood pressure elevated because of the vasospasm.

She told me that it would probably be around 110 and for me not to worry. When I told her that I saw it go up to about 125, she looked a little concerned and went in to check on him.

His sister Linda was beside the bed talking to him. The nurse looked at the monitor and then checked his pulse rate. She pulled me aside and told me that it could just be the fact that there was a lot of traffic and she would keep an eye on him. Again she told me not to worry.

After his family left, I went out into the courtyard. I sat down and cried, pondering over the events of the past few days. How could this be happening to him? What would I do if I ever lost him? I could not stop crying. It must have been a good hour of just sitting and crying before I could pull myself together and go back upstairs to him.

THURSDAY MAY 21, 1992

Blood type O+
Blood level is low
Two units of blood given
Lungs sound better
He is trying to lift his head
Must feel restraints – keeps trying to lift hands
Restraints tighter.
Temperature not above 101 degrees
Still on cooling blanket
Has opened his eyes two times for nurses during suctioning
They have to suction him every one to two hours
Finally, he opened his eyes for me

That's the day that I finally fell apart. I simply broke down. I cried because he would open his eyes for the nurses and not for me. I would cry because of the fever. Mostly I cried because he would lie there so helpless and there was nothing I could do for him. I didn't know how to help him. I felt as though I was losing something and I had no control over it.

The nurses asked me to sit and talk with the unit's neuro-psychologist. She was available to the patient's family and they thought that it might help me if I spoke to her.

I didn't want to. This place was for Steve. These doctor's were here to help Steve, not me. After a few minutes of arguments from the nurse, I agreed. The neurological psychologist was a very nice woman. She did her best to understand me, but I don't think I was making much sense. I told her how helpless I felt. How I felt that I was losing control of everything. We talked about the kids and how miserable I felt having to leave them at such a crucial time. She told me that I was where I should be. That my children were being well taken care of, and that right now my husband needed me more. She tried to explain to me that at times like this, sacrifices needed to be made. She said that the children, although troubled about everything right now, would be fine when it was all over.

Then she told me that if I didn't feel at times like I was out of control or had the helpless feelings that I have now that then she would be worried about me. What she didn't like was the fact that I was at the hospital all by myself while I was feeling like this. She asked me if she could call my mother. I told her not to and asked instead if she would simply let me call my sister. She nodded her head in agreement but reminded me that I shouldn't try to do this alone.

I went down to the lobby to use a pay phone and called Debbi. When she picked up the phone, I started sobbing.

"Laura, is Steve okay?" she asked.

"Debbi, he's fine. It's me. I think I'm falling apart." I quickly explained to her what the doctor had told me about wanting someone here with me. Debbi told me that she would be there as soon as she could.

I hung up the phone, went out to the courtyard and sat on the steps. I could not have been there for more than a half an hour when Debbi rushed up beside me, sat down and put her arm around me.

I started to cry uncontrollably. Everything was coming out all at once. It felt as though I had lost touch with the way I had been trying to handle things up until now.

"Debbi, I am so afraid of losing him. I am so afraid that if something does go wrong that he will leave me."

She looked at me with a puzzled expression in her eyes, "What do you mean, if something goes wrong? What happened?"

"Nothing happened. But he could still have a stroke. He really isn't coming around. What if something is wrong? If he does have a stroke or if he is paralyzed at all, he will leave me. He told me that a long time ago! He said that if he couldn't be a real husband to me, a real dad to the kids that it wasn't worth it." I must have sounded hysterical. I remembered a movie we had watched where the husband had been shot and was paralyzed from the waist down. "He's too proud of a man to stay with us in that condition!"

"Listen to me!" she said, "Steve is not going to leave you!" She turned me around and looked in my eyes. "He loves you. You and Steve will get through this. I know you will."

We talked for a long time and then she brought me into the cafeteria for something to eat. Then we went upstairs to see Steve. I arranged for Debbi to be allowed in to see him.

She told Steve how good he was doing. Then she told him to hang in there and left me alone with him.

I stood by his bed for about an hour. I couldn't talk to him. I just held his hand and silently let the tears run down my cheeks. I looked at his face and called his name. I couldn't believe it. He opened his eyes. Just for a moment but they opened. He seemed to be looking at me.

When I was getting ready to leave, a nurse took me by the arm. "Are you going to be okay?" she asked. She was concerned about me. Her name was Barbara. She was looking at my hands, they were shaking so bad that I could not stop them. She walked me over to a doctor.

"Dr. Pacsobann?" she started, "This is Mrs. Merrow. I think we should give her something to calm her down a little."

I protested. I told them that I didn't want anything to make me sleepy or that would put me out. I had to be able to be there for Steve.

They told me it would just be enough to relax me. I must have agreed with them because the next thing I knew one of them put a pill in my hand and the other was giving me something to wash it down with.

Al was waiting with my sister when I got back out to the waiting room. They brought me back to my parent's house. It was about an hour later that I got a phone call from a Doctor Shelito.

He said they were going to be surgically putting a tube into Steve's stomach. This would enable them to feed him and give him medication that would normally be taken by mouth.

I panicked. Was there something wrong? Was this being done tonight and did they need me to come back to the hospital?

The doctor on the other end of the phone sounded as if he were getting impatient with me. "Mrs. Merrow," he said, "the procedure won't be done until Tuesday. I am simply calling you to get a verbal consent and to answer any questions you may have."

Well I had a lot of questions. Most of them I wanted to ask Dr. Ogilvy. Which I did. I had him paged and he returned my call shortly after. I had been caught off guard. Maybe I was being a hysterical wife, but I needed some answers.

Dr. Ogilvy was very patient with me. He sounded as though he would have stayed on the phone with me for hours if he thought it would help to ease my mind.

Dr. Paul Shelito
It was called a G Tube
They would be going down his esophagus (similar to the way scope test is performed) with a microscope with a light on the end of it.
An incision would be made on the outside of the abdomen and then into the stomach
Risks: a low risk procedure
Perforation of the bowel / pneumonia / infection
Possibility of damage to the throat incision
The entire procedure only takes twenty minutes to a half an hour

The spasm he is having, is it on the main vessel to the brain and can it cause a massive stroke?
THERE IS NO WAY OF KNOWING WHAT CAN

HAPPEN, BUT THE SPASM IS ON THE MAIN VESSEL

Can the procedure on Tuesday irritate this spasm?
PROBABLY NOT BUT AGAIN, THERE IS NO WAY OF PREDICTING THESE THINGS

What if anything can he be told of what has happened?
EVERYTHING THAT I THINK HE CAN HANDLE. I KNOW HIM BEST
How do we know when the spasm stops?   *T H E ANGIOGRAM WOULD SHOW A LOT.*
Is he in pain?   *NOT   REALLY,   HE COULD BE HAVING A HEADACHE, BUT THE PAIN IS PROBABLY MINIMAL.*

I did not want the pill they had given me at the hospital, but after the phone call from Dr. Shelito, I guess it helped me to get the sleep that I so desperately needed. The next day I seemed to be a little bit more in control of myself.

FRIDAY MAY 22, 1992

Day nurse – Deborah
Responded during the night to simple commands
Opened eyes and squeezed Gail's hand.
Scheduled at one o'clock for an angiogram
He is awake.
Focusing
Can't vocalize, but is mouthing words
Fever still up.
Could be starting to break – he has the shakes
Nurses shaved his entire face during the night
Blisters were infected and the old blood in the beard was
impossible to clean. Mustache was irritating sores on lip.
Down to 40% oxygen.
Fever?
A possibility could be a blood spill into the brain stem itself.
When blood leaks from an aneurysm into the brain stem, it
can cause a high fever

Everyone is telling me that I am doing so great. To hang in there. That Steve is a strong man, a young man and that he would be fine. It didn't matter. I was waiting to hear those words from one person and one person only – Steve.

My parents each day made sure that I had enough to eat. That I was keeping up with my sleep. My father would come home from work at night and wait for me to call him to let him know that I wanted to leave the hospital. I didn't want to leave. What if he needed me for something?

I would call Steve's mother two or three times a day to let her know what was going on. She wanted to be at the hospital but was afraid of driving in Boston. His sister Linda was pregnant and due within the next month. She had been advised not to travel very far.

Each night when I got back to my parents house, I would call and talk to my children. Danielle, the oldest, knew exactly what was going on. She was amazing. When I called her at her Grandmothers that first day, I couldn't believe her response. I explained to her that there was something in Steve's brain that was leaking and that he was going to need to be operated on. She knew right away that it was an aneurysm. When I explained to her that it was being done in Boston at Mass. General, she also knew that it was very serious. So Danielle was kept informed of his condition every step of the way. She is a very intelligent girl. Sometimes though, I wished that she wasn't. This was an awful lot for an eleven year old to have to handle. She is a trooper though, she really is.

Jimmy at nine, understood that Steve was in serious condition but was too young to be told everything. I explained to him that while Steve was in the hospital there would be three stages. The first was while he was in I.C.U., the second would be when he was transferred to a regular unit and finally the third would be when he was sent to a rehabilitation hospital.

The rehabilitation hospital was not a definite at this point, but I needed the kids to be prepared for that. Dr. Ogilvy had told me that Steve may need anywhere from two to eight weeks in a rehabilitation facility. Everything depended on his recovery. At this point the doctor said is was an eighty percent chance that he would have to go.

Jimmy, each time we spoke, would ask what stage Steve was at. Right after surgery, he wanted to know what Steve looked like. The only way I could think of to describe it to him was that he looked like he had been in a fight. He had a black eye, of sorts, and a very fat lip. Jim thought that was okay, because the black eye would go away.

Dawn-dawn, as she had been nicknamed, was the tough one to talk to. Though I didn't want her to know too much, she still had to be told that her Daddy was in the hospital and would be there for quite some time. She had overheard enough that she knew he had been through an operation. She and I would end each conversation in the same manner. I would tell her that I loved her and she would give me a kiss over the phone and ask me to tell her Daddy that tomorrow he was going to have a "very good day!"

Then there would be the times when Becky would get on the phone and tell me hello over and over again. She is my heart breaker. Hearing her voice on the phone only made the longing for my children that much stronger. She is only a year and a half old but had the power to wrench every motherly instinct out of me. If only I could split myself in two and be in two places at one time.

I was where I had to be. The kids knew that and they really did understand. The way I explained it to Dawn was that she was at a place that had a lot of people who loved her very much. Her Daddy, however, even though the doctors and the nurses took very good care of him, needed to have someone there who loved him, too. She felt that it was a good idea then, for me to stay at her Nana and Papa's house so that I could be that someone for her Daddy.

My thoughts also went out to Steve's daughter, Andrea. She was only ten years old and must also be worried about her father. I called Florida to update her mother on what was going and Andrea answered the phone. I asked her if her mother had told her what was happening.

"Yes, she told me that Dad had to have an operation," she said.

"That's right. He is getting stronger and stronger every day. He will be okay, but it is going to take some time. He will probably be in the hospital for quite a while." I tried to reassure her of the fact that Steve would be okay. It was hard because I wasn't sure of how much she had been told.

I ended with asking her to have her mother call me if she had any questions, but that I would keep in touch.

I sat on the porch that night and thought about all the people that this was touching. Each one was being touched by it in a different way. Yet each one was relying on me to keep them informed and to be able to give them reassurance of some sort. It was starting to get harder and harder to perform both of those tasks.

SATURDAY MAY 23, 1992

A.M. nurse – Deborah
Fever at 102
Still the same as yesterday – no changes
Fever at one o'clock up to 104 degrees
On a cooling blanket top and bottom

The fever was scaring me. There was currently no answer to why he kept spiking a fever. Every possible test had been done to help them determine what was causing the infection. Someone told me that they might get the fever down and yet never know what had caused it.

My parents have told me that I can stay with them for as long as I need to. I only wish that I knew exactly how long that would be.

I look into his eyes and try to imagine what could possibly be going through his mind. I try to talk to him about the kids, but when I speak about Danielle or Jimmy he gets very upset. The only thing that the nurses and I can determine is that he may be thinking that the seizure hit him while he was still in the truck with the kids. Every time I bring them up or talk to him about them, he gets tears in his eyes and slams his fist down on the bed. I try to tell him that they are okay and at Linda's house. Oh I wish that I could get through to him.

My parents came in today to visit with him. I guess I really didn't prepare my mother for all the monitors and their alarms. As soon as she walked into his room, an alarm on both his blood pressure monitor and the respirator went off. Not only that but the alarm on his IV monitor started to beep as well. During all of this, two people from radiology came in to take an x-ray of his lungs. They were pushing a portable x-ray machine.

My mother thought that all the commotion was due to her coming into the room. She turned around apologizing to me, then with tears in her eyes she fled back down to the waiting room.

I followed her out. I tried to reassure her that it was nothing terrible and that it had nothing to do with her going into the room. I told her that he was going to be okay, but I knew that a lot of her anxiety was my fault. I should have prepared her more than I had.

I had asked the doctor to sit with me and go over the different tests that they had given Steve. I wanted to see the CT-scans, angiogram and the M.R.I. that had been done prior to the operation. Dr. Ogilvy thought that was fine and arranged to be at the hospital at around seven o'clock to sit with me.

That day was so long. Steve was awake off and on, trying his best to communicate with me. By the end of the day I was totally drained. The nurses thought I should call it a day. I looked at the clock and say that it was only five thirty. They were right. I would never make it until seven. I asked that they please get in touch with the doctor and let him know that I was leaving the hospital.

That night when I called to check on Steve, a nurse told me that the doctor had been there with a file full of x-rays to go over with me. I felt so guilty. Yet I had asked that someone let him know that I would not be there. She told me that the nursing staff did not call him or his office unless it was an emergency. She said that I could call him anytime however if I needed him, but that they could not.

That is how I found out exactly who Dr. Ogilvy was. He was the professor of neuro-surgery at Mass General and considered one of the tops in his field in the country. When he was not in the operating room then he could be found doing research. He was an extremely important surgeon. The best they had.

SUNDAY MAY 24, 1992

A.M. nurse – Deborah
Awake and very agitated
Skin graft scared him
Temperature down to 102 to 103 degrees
Vision to the left in the left eye paralyzed
8 to 10 weeks to regain
Spoke to anesthesia doctor for consent for Tuesdays
surgical procedure
Will it be done in his room or in the operating room?
IN THE OPERATING ROOM
Saw Dr. Ogilvy. He went over the CT-scans angiograms
and the MRI with me

Steve's mother came to the hospital tonight to visit with her friend Tom. She got in to see Steve a couple of times. However, because of his fever and the blister on his lip that was weeping, she really didn't want to kiss him. He made up for it though. Even though he couldn't talk, he looked at her when she was saying her good-byes and blew her a kiss. It melted her heart. I am sure that she will remember that for the rest of her life.

Afterwards, I sat with Al, his mother and Tom and explained to them what my consultation with the doctor was about.

The fact that his fever is so high was the main concern right now. There was also a very bad pressure blister on his upper lip and it was weeping. This was caused from the equipment used on his mouth during the surgery. I had been asked that each time I touched his face or kissed him to clean with an alcohol wipe. The nurses always made sure that there was a good supply on hand.

Doctor Ogilvy had shown me exactly where the leak had come from. The operation had been very successful but where they had been working was very close to the nerves of the left eye. The doctor pointed this out to me on the angiogram. He was hopeful that the nerve was simply in shock or possibly that it was traumatized. He was also very hopeful that his vision would be totally regained in about eight to ten weeks.

Most of what he was trying to explain escapes me now, but I will always remember the x-rays and the films that he showed to me. I was in total amazement. This thing, this aneurysm, was right in the center of Steve's brain.

I had so many things go through my mind. This could have happened at home. It could have happened while he was, God forbid, driving his truck that morning with everyone in it. Worst of all, it could have happened while we were on vacation, on a boat, in the middle of the ocean while we were deep-sea fishing.

So, the good Lord, in His infinite wisdom, must have been watching over Steve. If this was going to have to happen, at least it happened where it did, and he was taken care of promptly.

So I explained all of this to them. By the time I was finished, I could tell that they all had a lot of questions. Especially from his mother. I tried to answer every question as best and as fully as I possibly could. They needed to understand what was happening to Steve. I wanted them to know how grave and serious this was. How lucky he had been to get this far but that he still had a long way to go.

I explained to them about Steve's eye and what the doctor had told me. It seemed that every time I tried explaining one thing it would be followed by another flood of questions. My mind was spinning, searching for the right words to say. I wanted to be able to give some comfort to his mother but I also had to tell her the truth about everything. I was so in need of the comfort I was so patiently giving.

So many times during the explanations I had to stop and catch my breath. I wanted to just break down and cry. Al went down to the first floor and brought me a bottle of apple juice. I thanked him, took a sip and said my good byes to Steve's mother and Tom. I wanted to go in to say good night to Steve before Al had to bring me back to my parent's house. His mother gave me a hug and told me to give Steve her love.

I walked to the intercom and buzzed the nurse's station for permission to be let back in. I could hear the muffled voices coming from the waiting room. I was hoping that what I had told them had been understood. I wanted so badly for them to understand. I didn't know if I could explain everything all over again.

Steve's mother was planning to come in the next day to visit with him. Tom had the day off because it was Memorial Day. However after she left that night, the nurses and the doctor talked to me about Steve's fever.

That was his biggest enemy right now, they said. Any other type of infection would only cause it to escalate. They were very concerned that germs being carried in off of the street would be transmitted to him. They wanted the family and I to be aware of this problem. A possibility of gloves and a mask was mentioned. The bottom line came down to them requesting that until his fever was under control that visiting should be limited to his wife.

I had to call his mother and let her know. I would do it in the morning. Her visit with Steve had gone so well that I couldn't tell her this tonight. Instead I called his older sister. I definitely thought she should know though, because she was pregnant.

The next morning I called his mother. After explaining to her what they had said, I told her about the visiting limitation that had been put into effect.

I promised that I would call each day and at night to let her know what was happening.

I felt so alone.

I hung up the telephone, wishing and praying that the day would bring good news. That somehow, I would get to the hospital and have this horrible mess over with. But I knew that I was fantasizing. That this was real.

I had sat with my mother before she left for work over a cup of coffee, and told her the events of the night before.

She was so helpful. She reminded me that Steve had gotten through the surgery. That he was getting better and better each and every day. For me not to lose hope. Not to let the concerns about his fever get to me. That with Steve's strong will and my constant vigil, we would be okay.

She got herself ready for work. As she was leaving she turned around and came back to me with a big hug and a kiss.

"You hang in there," she said.

"I have to Mom, I have to for Steve." I kissed her on the cheek and told her to have a good day. She told me to do the same, and to send Steve her love.

MONDAY MAY 25, 1992

It was Al's day off from the store so he had come down to take me in to the hospital. He stayed in the waiting room while I went in to see Steve. I buzzed the nurse's station from the intercom outside the unit.

"Deborah will be out to get you in a moment," it answered when I asked if I could come in to see Steve.

A moment later Deborah met me at the door. She said that she wanted to talk to me before I went to see him. "He is very confused," she said. "He is unaware of where he is or why he is even here." She went on to tell me that it was very normal after surgery involving the brain. It was a temporary condition and it would come and go.

I told her that I understood and asked her what I should do. She told me that I would know at the time. To simply change the subject or to even leave the room if he got too upset.

I walked into the room and as always, the first thing that I did was to check his vital signs on the monitors. Everything was looking good. Everything that is, except his temperature. That was still high.

He started to stir. I grabbed his hand and said, "Good morning, honey!"

He looked at me and pulled his hand from mine. He was looking me square in the face and was mouthing some words. I couldn't make them out at first and asked him to go slower. The next time it was quite clear what he was trying to say.

"Where is my wife?"

I felt my throat tighten. "Steve it's me!"

He shook his head and his mouth started moving again. "Go and find my wife, you bitch." Then he closed his eyes.

I felt Deborah come up behind me. I turned around. She grabbed my shoulders and looked at me. "What's wrong?" she asked.

"He...he doesn't know who I am!" I replied. I couldn't control the tears.

She guided me of the room. "I told you that he was confused" she said. "I told you that this could happen."

"It would not have mattered," I was sobbing. "You could have given me something in writing. It could have been in black and white that on this day, at this time he would look at me and not know who I was. It just wouldn't have mattered. It would have still hurt." I pulled myself away from her and ran. I ran right out of the double doors of the unit. I was crying hysterically. I went right past the waiting room and pushed the button for the elevator. I pushed it again and again, as though pushing it would get the doors to open quicker. I could hear Al walking and then running to catch up with me. He was as white as a ghost. He must have thought that something was wrong with Steve. "He's okay!!" I shouted. The tears kept coming. I kept banging at the elevator button. "He is okay. He just doesn't know me! He doesn't know who I am!"

The elevator doors opened, and Al ushered me in. He took me down to the courtyard and sat me at a table while he went to get me a cup of coffee. While he was gone I managed to pull myself back together. I was so angry with myself. I had promised myself that I would not let Steve see me cry. It was just that it hurt so much.

I was told today that when they were putting Steve in the ambulance at the store, that he was yelling "Don't let me die!"

Each day that passes I will be that much stronger.
I need to be strong for him. I need to be able to be with him.

Dear God, You've given him back to me, now please give me the strength to see him through the rest

I managed to get enough strength to go back into his room. This time he knew who I was. He was still confused about where he was. When I asked him if he understood what had happened to him, he just shook his head no. I tried to slowly tell him. I asked if he remembered the headaches. He nodded. I told him that there had been an aneurysm leaking inside his head. His hand pulled up on the restraint. I loosened it for him and guided his hand to the splint on his nose and the bandage on his head and face. I let him feel the trachea. I explained that it was not going to be there for that long, that it was not permanent, that was why he couldn't speak though.

I looked into his eyes. He was crying. I tried to reinforce with him that the kids were fine. That this had not happened in the truck. He nodded his head and then closed his eyes and fell back to sleep.

I put his hand back down on the bed and replaced the restraint. The nurse came in and I told her that I was better, and that Steve seemed to understand what I had said. She told me to be ready to repeat the entire story to him tomorrow.

Doctor Ogilvy was at the nurse's station when I was leaving and asked me if he could speak with me. I nodded and he walked with me to a conference room. I wanted to ask him about the confusion, but he stopped me. He began talking about the way his blood pressure and heart rate skyrocketed whenever visitors passed through his room. He was getting concerned and wanted to discuss it with me.

He hesitated and then went on to explain that as far as the fever was concerned, the partial quarantine was one thing but that a full restriction on visitors was not in their powers. He told me that they were still watching the vaso-spasm. That Steve was still in danger of having a stroke. Whenever his blood pressure went up so did his chances of having a stroke. Now that his confusion was present and as strong as it was, it also presented a problem. Where I was with him constantly, I had learned to work with it and learned how to handle Steve with it. Others wouldn't have that advantage. The more confused Steve got, the harder it would be for visitors to understand him. The harder it was for him to be understood, the more aggravated he got. The more aggravated he got, the higher his blood pressure went. It was a very dangerous circle. It was one symptom feeding and upsetting the other.

He asked me how I felt about everything. I told him that I had informed his family and mine that for the next four days the only one that would be allowed in would be me, but that it was because of the fever. He told me that the confusion would probably go on longer than that. I turned around and sat down to think.

"I could tell them it will take longer, but I don't know how long I can do that. I can't tell his family that their presence in front of Steve will pose a threat to his life. They are all going through enough hell right now"

I looked up at the doctor. "I'll tell them something. I have to."

He nodded his understanding. Other than the confusion, which was to be expected, and the fever, Doctor Ogilvy seemed very encouraged with Steve's progress. He also told me that he was very concerned that I was not taking good care of myself. He said that I had to be careful and to keep up with my sleep and my eating habits.

He patted me on the back and told me to hang in there. He seemed to say that to me a lot. It seemed like such a simple phrase. Who would know that I would grow to hate those words? That each time he said them to me, they would sting my heart and pierce my soul.

TUESDAY MAY 26, 1992

A.M. nurse Cheryl
Doing fine – no changes
Temperature at 101 degrees (still)
Scheduled: CT Scan
Ventriculostomey (new drain)
G-tube – surgery
P.M. Steve was alert but concerned and scared
On a double catheter – (urine catheter and a rectal bag
Because of the diarrhea)
Saw Dr. Ogilvy again – still encouraged with Steve's progress

They had to change the drain on his head because it was in for too many days. Something about after fourteen days with it on it had to be changed to prevent infection.

The surgery with Dr. Shelito went fine. It was not done until after I had left. The doctor called me at home that night to let me know that it was over and that he was fine.

I called his family and let them know that he was okay and that the surgery was over. Then I called Linda Grant and spoke with the kids.

My parents are concerned about me. They are afraid that I am not taking care of myself. I told them it didn't matter how I was. I knew what they meant though. They only wanted to protect me as parents are supposed to.

I tried to explain to them that I was not the issue. Steve was. That I was only doing what I had to do for Steve.

They told me the same thing. They only wanted me to take care of myself in order to be able to care for Steve.

WEDNESDAY MAY 27, 1992

A.M. nurse – Cheryl
Temperature still at 101 degrees

Met Dr. Gress (in charge of I.C.U.) he passed me in the hall
while I was waiting to get in to see Steve.
He wanted to make sure that I was okay and that I was
keeping up with my rest and strength.

Met with Meredith – a social worker I think. She just
listened to me babble and babble. What I need to do is just
hold on to the fact that he is alive.

Each decision I've made has been harder than the one before.
I know that Steve will be okay. She spoke to me about the
visitors being restricted.
She has gone over Steve's medical record and tended to agree
with the Doctor and with me. If it helped matters, she said
she would talk to the family for me.

Steve, I've been so afraid to write down how scared I
am. Everyone has been so good to me and the nursing staff
has been so patient, too. I feel so lost when I am not at the
hospital. I know that each day you face the same fears as
the day before. I wish I could hold you and tell you not to be
afraid. But who wouldn't be?

It's warmer today. I sit in the courtyard and try to picture
you sitting out here with the kids.
Soon.

PM May 27th

Spoke with Dede
She is amazed at Steve's condition and the fact that he is
doing so well.
Temperature is down to 99.8 degrees.
Very tired from yesterday.
Neck very stiff.
Still breathing on his own, with very minimal support.
Swelling on lip is going down.
Legs not restrained any longer.
Changed his antibiotics during the day.

THURSDAY MAY 28, 1992

The sun's up and I hope it stays out.
Weatherman says the next few days will be nice.
70 – 75 through Saturday. It will make for a nice day with
the kids on Saturday.
I keep waking up looking for you.

A.M. nurse – Cheryl
Ninth day since surgery.
Twelfth day in the hospital
Temperature up to 101 degrees (not higher than 102 during
the night)
No changes.
May have a follow up CT scan today.

Questions for the doctor:
How much longer in I.C.U.? ***HOPING FOR EARLY***
TO MIDDLE OF NEXT WEEK.
How much longer with the trachea? ***COUPLE OF***
WEEKS.
How long will the G-tube be in? ***LONGER THAN***
THE TRACHEA.
Any answers to the fever yet? ***NONE YET***
How is the nose and sinus cavity healing? ***L O O K S***
GOOD

Caught the bus at 9:21 this morning
Steve would probably not like me taking the bus, but he

could think of it this way. I'm saving money and not driving around Boston by myself.

I sit again in the courtyard. Somehow, just being here I feel relaxed. I am closer to you.

I close my eyes at night and know that you have made it through another day. One step closer to coming home.

I need so badly to have you come back to me Steve.

It tears me apart knowing how terrified you must be each morning. Not knowing if you can comprehend what has happened. Each day that passes I am realizing just how close I came to losing you.

But I didn't Steve.

Just keep fighting.

Each day it's the same thing. Catch the bus, catch the train. Call his mother, call his sister, call Linda. Remind him that he is at Mass. General. Reassure him that it's going to be okay. That he is going to be fine.

I sit in the waiting room and watch the families' come and go. I never thought I would know what it would feel like to be able to know what they are going through. The worst feeling is when you don't see them anymore. You wonder what happened. Sometimes you know that something had to have gone wrong with their family member. They just weren't there long enough.

MAY 28th – P.M.

Will probably be taken off the ventilator completely after the CT scan.

Fever down to 99.8 degrees with Tylenol

*Cheryl is talking about physical therapy. I will have to get
him some high top sneakers.
Deborah will be on at 3:00
Steve left the floor at 2:08 for the CT Scan*

Each time Steve left the floor there would be a nurse that
went with him. It tore me up inside watching them transport
him. Due to the fact that he was on the respirator, they would
have to "bag" him during the trip. I had a fear of whoever it
was that pumped the bag that kept Steve breathing, tripping or
missing a breathe.

I couldn't sit in the waiting room any more. It was heart
breaking to watch a new family going through the misery I had
experienced. So I would sit at the end of the corridor. There
was a wall made of glass windows with a ledge to sit on. There
I would sit...and wait. I would usually have a book opened, but
very rarely did I see the words. Only the corridor. I would wait
for the elevator doors to open and a stretcher to come off with
Steve on it, back from some procedure. In either case that
small bit of ledge in front of the glass became the place I will
remember the most. Dr. Gress laughingly referred to it as my
"office".

FRIDAY MAY 29, 1992

They all wonder how I can stay at the hospital for as long as I do.
They wonder how, but they never wonder why. It is so difficult
to explain. There are so many nights that I am lucky to get an
hour or two of sleep, yet I have the strength to face yet another
long and grueling day of emotional ups and downs.

My mother is so relieved that I am spending the weekend
with the children. She knows that emotionally I am completely
drained. This will give me a diversion away from everything.

A.M nurse Cheryl
Temperature still down at 98.6 degrees!
Off the ventilator – doing all his own breathing.
Very antsy

12:00 NOON...
Doing great – looks good.
Blood pressure alarm reduced – down to 150/170 (the top
number from 160/180
Heart rate is between 85-90
Oxygen – 100% saturated.

He is feeling his head, the stitches, his nose.

He has a headache.
Sleepy
Questions for the doctor:
How long on seizure medication?   ***ON***

PHENOBARBITAL FOR ABOUT 6 MONTHS TO A YEAR

Chances of recurring seizures?   **NO WAY OF KNOWING.**

The worst part of the day is when I first show up in the hospital, I normally have to wait for about a half an hour to see Steve.

Watching his anger excites and terrifies me at the same time.

I was so happy to see him fighting the restraints and wanting to pull at the tubes, but at the same time I was scared of him hurting himself and having a set back.

He has come so far to have anything happen now.

I need to talk to Dr Tatta

Just being able to sit and be in his room feels so good. I watch everything, the monitors the IV's and his chest.

Watching his chest is so good. Each time it expands on its own, I know he is on his way back.

I wish I could read his mind. More than that I wish I could read his lips.

I stayed with him all day. Tomorrow I will not be here. I am leaving tonight to go home and see the kids. It has been two weeks since this entire nightmare began and they needed me. I needed them too. Needed to hold them and feel their love. Needed to let them know that it was going to be okay. Needed to let me know that they were okay.

I tried my best to explain this to him. I don't think he really heard me. He slept most of the day. I would sit in a chair in the corner of the room and just watch him.

The nurses have been so good to me. They realize that we have a special closeness. They know that I am strong and that I am not bothered by them changing a dressing or suctioning out his trachea. They have let me stay in his room for up to an hour or so at a time. I leave when I think that I am in their way or to simply get a breath of fresh air.

I decided to take pictures of all the kids while I was at home for him. I especially wanted to get a good shot of both Danielle and Jimmy so that I could show him that they were okay.

They are talking about getting him out of the bed and putting him into what is called a cardiac chair. This chair lies flat up against his bed. They will slide him onto it and then crank it into an upright position.

It broke my heart to leave that night. I knew it would only be for one day. I was planning on being back here first thing on Sunday morning. But it just hurt me so much to leave. When it was time to go, I woke him up and reassured him that I would only be gone for tomorrow and that I would be checking in with the nurses to make sure that he was okay. If he needed me to be there for anything, someone would call me. I gave him a kiss and went out the door. As the tears flowed down my cheeks, I knew that a part of me was still in that room. I left my heart at his bedside.

Al was waiting for me downstairs and drove me home. When we got there it was after 11:00 and my friend Linda was waiting for me. I put my arms out to her and we held on to each other for quite a long time. We had always tried to be there for the other. At that moment, I needed her to hold me. I needed to feel safe.

We sat and talked until about two o'clock in the morning. Even when she left, I felt her with me. I checked in on all the kids to be sure they were all sleeping.

That night was going to take forever to end. I walked into my bedroom. It was obvious that no one had been there since I left. The bed was still unmade with the suitcase opened, waiting to be packed for our vacation. I put it aside and went back out to the kitchen. I couldn't stay in there. I started to cry. It seemed like it had been an eternity since I had been here. I felt so alone in my own house. I went back to the bedroom, grabbed a pillow and tried to sleep on the couch. It wasn't helping. After about an hour of tossing and turning, I swallowed my fears and went back to my bedroom.

I must have lied there for hours. The tears would not stop, but they washed me into a restless sleep. A sleep I was gratefully awakened from early in the morning by a scuffling of feet out in the kitchen. It was Dawn. I went out to the kitchen. Dawn took one look at me and jumped into my arms. We went in to get Becky up and within minutes all four children were around my feet.

We had a wonderful day. Sue came by to give me a hand. We all went shopping for a get-well card and a present for Daddy. They decided on a Teddy Bear that had legs and arms that bent. That way he could sit on Daddy's bedside table. Their Grammy, Steve's mom, stopped by to visit with them later that day and we all sat around and had a pizza party.

SATURDAY MAY 30, 1992

Throughout the entire day I was constantly calling the hospital to check on Steve. I needed to know that he was okay.

No major changes
Temperature is still down
Told nurse, Barbara, to put on channel 25 so that Steve could watch his wrestling.
Called later to check on him.
Doing fine – watching wrestling

I wish I could be there
I am so glad I'm here

The kids are great.
Took them to Ames to buy Steve a get-well card and a present.
Questions for the doctor:
How is he tolerating the feeding tube? **TOLERATED THE FEEDING FINE. NO PROBLEMS**
Did they get him in a chair? **PUT IN A CARDIAC CHAIR. SAT UP, SLOUCHED SOME, BUT WAS ABLE TO REPOSITION HIMSELF FINE**
Barbara tried to keep him awake and interested in the television during the day. Temperature at night still fine

SUNDAY MAY 31, 1992

Although the time spent with the kids was terrific, I still felt so lost. So all alone. I knew I had to be back with him. Sunday morning came. I cooked the kids a special breakfast. I wanted so badly to be able to be in two places at one time, here and at the hospital.

Linda's husband Robert was at the house to get the kids by nine o'clock as promised. He sat down at the kitchen table and Becky went over and jumped up in his lap. He took one look at me and knew that if he didn't get the kids out of there he was going to have not only crying children on his hands but that I would be crying as well. I gave each one of them a hug and a kiss as I watched them leave.

It wasn't until they were out of earshot that I broke down in tears. As much as it tore me up inside to leave them, I knew where I had to be. I knew I had to get back to the hospital.

> *Back at the hospital by ten thirty this morning.*
> *Hard watching the kids leave in the morning, but they will be fine*
> *Steve needs me and they know that.*
> *Steve sat in the cardiac chair again while I was in the room. He wanted to get up and walk. Body still too weak.*
> *Spoke to Dr. Ogilvy. Steve is doing very well. He is saying that now we have to watch the incision in the back of his throat. Has to be sure that there is not any leakage. Scheduled Steve for a test on Tuesday.*
> *Very confused off and on during the day. Has not needed any valium though so far.*

Temperature still below 100 degrees. Moving more.
Playing mind games with the nurses. Trying to get them
angry.
Not talking to them

Steve's mother came in to see him. When she walked over to his bed to say hello to him, he put his arms out to her. It looked like he was trying to get her to hug him. So that was what she did. What she didn't know was that he was attempting the only way he knew to have her help him out of the bed.

It was also very frustrating to him when we could not understand what he was trying to say to us. I had not seen him this aggravated since he was operated on. The nurse came in and gave him a shot of valium. Then she asked that we leave the room for about a half an hour so that he would calm down.

I went out to the waiting room with his mother. We sat there for about forty minutes before the nurse, Barbara, came back to get us.

When I got back to his room, I couldn't believe what I saw. Steve had an iron-leveling bar in his hand and was about to swing it at one of the nurses as she had her back to him.

"STEVE!!" I screamed. "Knock it off. Put it down NOW!"

He dropped the level and looked at his mother and me. His mouth was moving, but I could not understand what he was trying to say. He was pointing at his mother, so she went to the head of his bed.

"I'm here," she was saying. Then tried to comfort him. She was trying to understand what it was that he was trying so desperately to say. He only got more and more agitated. The nurse left the room and came back in with another needle.

"What is that you're giving him now?" I asked. I couldn't understand what was going on. I looked at his monitors. His blood pressure was rising as well as his pulse. His heart rate was up to 120. It was too high.

The nurse looked at me and I could tell she was upset. "This is morphine. I need to calm him down." She was shaking her head. "I am going to have to ask the two of you to say your good nights to him." She looked at me and then at his mother. "Right now!"

Barbara went to the other side of the bed and gave him the shot of morphine. I watched her; she didn't like what she was seeing on the monitors or Steve's constant frustration. I nudged his mother out of my way and moved up to the head of the bed.

"We have to leave," I told him. "I will be back first thing in the morning." I gave him a kiss and said good night. I turned to his mother, "It's time to go. The nurse wants us to leave."

"I just want to say good night to him," she said. She moved up to the head of his bed.

"Mom," I said, "We have to leave right now." She said good night and I walked with her back to the waiting room. I looked at my purse and realized that I had left my notebook back in his room. I told Al that I would be right back out. I turned around and went back in to the unit.

Barbara was at the nurse's station. I went into Steve's room and grabbed my notebook. She was at the door and I could tell by the look on her face that she was about to remind me that she had asked me to leave.

"Barbara," I said, "What happened in there? Why did his vitals go up like that?" What bothered me more than that was that in the course of an hour he had needed both valium and morphine. He hadn't needed anything like that all day.

"Listen," she said, "I haven't been with him that much. But I saw enough tonight to see that having new faces enter this room is upsetting him. Anyone other than his day-to-day nurses and you are getting him going. He sees them as someone else to work on. Someone new to get him out of that bed!"

I turned around and looked at Steve. The morphine had taken effect. He was sleeping. "What are you trying to say?" I asked her.

"I can't say anything. I can only tell you what is happening to my patient. You are here everyday. You know how to react to his confusion." She paused and looked at me as though she were fighting with her thoughts and words.

"Mrs. Merrow," she said, "If I were you, I would take a real close look at the situation, his condition and his reactions. You are the only one who can impose any restrictions on his visitors."

I didn't know what to say. I listened to her telling me how people who could not properly deal with the confusion will only cause it to worsen. The more agitated he became because someone either didn't understand what he was saying or what he meant because of the fact that he was confused, the worse the confusion would become.

I understood what she was saying. The only thing was that it was a lot easier said than done.

How in Heavens name was I going to explain to his family that they would not be allowed in to see him? She suggested that I talk it over with the social worker assigned.

I felt so damn helpless. The nurse was right. It wasn't going to matter who it was. Steve wanted out of the bed. He wanted the monitors and the IV lines off. What was I going to do?

When I got back to my parents house, I sat and explained to my mother what was going on. She said the decision was mine, that it was his family though, and his mother. I had to find a way to do this so that Steve would be able to stay calm and safe, and his family would be able to understand. If they ever could. How could I do this? Dear God, help me to make the right decision.

I lie awake all night trying to piece together what it was that I had to do. The most important thing of all was Steve. I had to do what was best for him. I had to do everything I could to keep him calm. To keep him alive. He was still in danger of having a stroke because of the vasospasm. If his blood pressure kept going up it would only make matters that much worse.

One of the nurses had told me she was very surprised at the amount of visiting traffic that went in and out of Steve's room. She told me that normally in I.C.U., the only one that usually saw a patient in critical condition was the spouse.

I guess that I knew what I had to do. I was going to have to put the families' feelings aside and concentrate on Steve. If the nurses felt that strongly about it then they must have a lot of concern over his well-being. I was torn between a rock and a hard place, as Steve would say. I was damned if I did and damned if I didn't. In my heart though, I knew I had no choice.

MONDAY JUNE 1, 1992

I sat with my coffee for almost an hour before I got the strength to start making my phone calls. I began with my sisters. After them, I called Steve's sister Linda.

I poured myself another cup of coffee and dialed the last number, his mother. It was going to be the hardest call I had ever made. It really hurt me to tell her.

To everyone else but my parents this was a decision made by the hospital. I couldn't tell anybody that it had been my ultimate decision. At this point, it only made sense to say the decision had been made by someone else. Someone with authority at the hospital. I couldn't afford for anybody to be upset right now. I had to keep things calm. For everybody concerned. It was the only way I knew of to do this.

There were no words that I could think of to explain to anybody that their presence was causing Steve's blood pressure to go sky high. It sounded so selfish to say that I was the only one allowed to see him. Everybody wanted the same thing that I did. We all wanted to see Steve through this horrible ordeal. I was so afraid that if the visitors didn't stop, like the nurses said, that Steve would get worse.

I had to promise his mother over and over again that I would keep in constant contact with her every day. That I would keep her up to date with everything that was going on.

I got off the phone and simply collapsed down to the floor and cried. I felt isolated. Now I would have to do it alone. There wouldn't be anybody to come in and give me a break. I only hoped the Lord would see fit to help me. To guide me to an answer.

I got myself together and headed to the hospital. When I got there, Steve was awake and sitting in his cardiac chair. I knelt down next to him and looked into his eyes. I told him everything. The truth of the past forty-eight hours. I put my head down on his lap and cried. When I looked back up at him he was nodding as if in agreement. His hands motioned down to his lap. Steve had only been wearing a towel or a blanket draped across his midsection while in I.C.U. His mouth was moving in a desperate attempt to say something. The best the nurses and I could come up with was to please save his dignity. He went on as if to tell us that he really didn't want anyone to see him in such a weak condition.

My heart broke for him. He was trying his best to ask me to save what little pride he had left. I told him not to worry, that I would take care of him. Maybe the restriction on the visitors was for the best. Steve wanted to get himself back on his feet first. Now I knew that I had made the right decision. I only hoped that his family would understand.

Rainy day!
Temperature still down.
A.M. nurse – Janice
In cardiac chair most of the morning.
Tried to get up out of the chair when the nurses were not there.

Taken off medication to regulate blood pressure.
At that time the first number was about 145 to 150. It went up to about 180 over 80. Had to be put back on the medication to lower it.

Probability of having blood pressure problem before being admitted.

Spoke with Dr. Mulligan. She is an occupational therapist. She showed me how to help exercise his arms and hands while he is in bed and while he is asleep.

Steve slept most of the day.

Spoke with Meredith, the social worker, she will check to see if we can get him into the rehab at Salem, N.H.
She will find out which ones are covered by Bay State Insurance.

She agreed with me, and my decision on the visitors. Said she was available to the family members as well as myself.
The restriction will probably hold until the family has spoken to Meredith or until he is out of I.C.U.

Tuesday JUNE 2, 1992

The test that is going to be performed today is very important. It is called a cisternogram. A dye would be injected into the lower portion of Steve's spine.

The dye would travel up the spinal column and enter his brain. Once there, a CT-scan would be performed. This procedure would enable them to know if there was any type of leakage around the area where the graft had been done.

In order to do this however, they had to remove all the packing from inside his nose. I was told the procedure would take the entire radiology team to do the cisternogram. They would need to turn him in different positions. The CT-scan would have to be done with him lying flat on his stomach. It would take anywhere from two to four hours.

When I got to the hospital and upstairs to his room, my heart jumped. He looked so good lying there with no bandages on his face. With the packing out, the look of swelling on his face was now gone. He was sitting up and smiling when I saw him. My Steve was a sight for sore eyes.

As always, I started my visit out by asking him where he was. I had to remind him which hospital he was in. I went through the same points with him. He was going to be all right. He had undergone an operation, which had saved his life, I told him. The kids were fine. Most importantly, I had to let him know that he was going to be fine.

Not all of what I said would be accepted. He sometimes didn't know or believe that he was in a hospital. The nurses would keep reassuring me that it was normal. They said it was very common and was referred to as "I.C.U. psychosis".

When the confusion hit him I tried my best to ride it out. I would either let it go, or try and help him understand. It was not easy to do since he couldn't talk to me.

He wanted me to find his suitcase. I kept trying to tell him that I hadn't brought one for him. Yet he was insistent that he had brought a suitcase. I would go on to tell him that an ambulance brought him here and then I would try to tell him that I hadn't brought the suitcase. He would get agitated, so I would let it be. I told him not to worry about it.

It wasn't always like that though. Most of the time he was alert. As alert as I could hope for, I guess.

A.M. nurse – Barbara
Cisternogram to performed today.
Packing to be removed from nose

Test went from 12:30 to 4:00
There is some leakage

They will be taking him to Mass. Eye and Ear tomorrow
To have some sutures put in.
Should help the confusion to go away.

Looks great with the bandages off.

Barbara went with him for the test.
Said the A-line came off during the cisternogram
Dr. Rafferty replaced it afterward.

Spoke with Dr. Ogilvy at night
Neurologically Steve is fine
Will need sutures to stop leakage
Doesn't sound overly concerned, but has to be done tomorrow.

I waited for Steve on the floor, outside the elevator doors in my "office". I would jump for every person that walked by. I could hear the elevator approaching the floor. When it opened, I saw his nurse, Barbara, getting off first. She pulled on the stretcher and I was stunned when I saw Steve. He was lying face down on the stretcher.

I waited for about fifteen minutes before trying to get in to see him. Barbara came out to greet me and go over what she had observed. He did fine during the test. She explained how during the test the A-line had come undone and that it was off now. She wasn't sure but felt that maybe he could go without it.

Having the A-line off would have been great; it was one thing that drove Steve crazy. The A-line was an IV line that went directly into a main artery instead of a vein. However later on that afternoon, Dr. Rafferty replaced it.

I asked Barbara what she thought about the test. She said she knew that there was a small leak on the preliminary reading, and she wasn't sure how they would repair it.

I spoke with Dr. Ogilvy that night. He said that they were going to try and repair the leak by going through the mouth. He told me that they would try to simply put a few sutures in the area that was leaking. However, he was not sure if they would be able to reach it that way. If they couldn't, they were going to have to reopen the original incision and get to it that way.

My heart dropped. Reopen?? How could Steve possibly endure yet another surgery? The doctor went on to explain that it would all be done at Mass. Eye and Ear. The instruments there were more delicate and Dr. Joseph, who would be the main surgeon, wanted it performed there.

Dr. Ogilvy would be assisting in the procedure. He told me that it would take a few hours. I was shaking, and unaware that there were tears streaming down my face.

The doctor reached over and handed me a tissue. He told me not to panic. This would be a minor operation compared to what he had already been through. He meant well, but his words were of little comfort to me at this point.

He finished up by telling me that it would be done tomorrow. They wouldn't be sure which way it would be done until they were underway. I would have no way of knowing until it was all over.

WEDNESDAY JUNE 3, 1992

When I arrived at the hospital I met his nurse Barbara on the elevator. She told me she was glad that she bumped into me before I saw Steve. He was alert and understood the fact that he was going to have the surgery done.

"Surgery?!?, I asked. " When was it confirmed that it would be surgery? What the hell happened to trying a couple of sutures first?"

She told me to calm down. "Either way, it will be necessary to put him to sleep."

The doors to the elevator opened but Barbara held me back and hit the button for the first floor. "Let's go outside and give you a chance to get yourself together before you see him."

She was right as usual. We got to the first floor and she went out to the courtyard with me and sat with me for a little while.

"Listen, don't quote me, but I think you ought to know this." She lit herself a cigarette and went on, "I am just going by my own past experience, but my opinion is that they are going to have to reopen him. I don't think you should be misled. You need to be prepared for what you are going to have to deal with. They will try to keep it to just a suture, but from what I read in his chart, I don't think it will happen. You are a strong lady and I know you can handle the truth about this."

Barbara hadn't pulled any punches with me so far. I knew in my heart that she wasn't doing that now. She told me that she would let me stay with Steve for as long as I wanted to. For as long as he needed me with him.

I listened to her as she told me how she noticed him

watching her this morning. How she explained to him what was going on. She wasn't sure how much he understood, but she was pretty sure he understood, and she was pretty sure he understood about the operation.

I took a deep breath and thanked her. Then I headed upstairs to Steve. I didn't know how to handle this. With everything he had already been through, he was never aware of what was happening until it was all over.

I smiled and gave him a kiss when I got to his bedside. "Good morning sweetheart." I released his hand restraints, as always, and held onto his hand. "Barbara told me that you know about the procedure today."

I could see in his eyes that he was alert, as Barbara had told me. He was frightened, too. He nodded his head and squeezed my hand tighter. His mouth started to go in an attempt to talk.

"Slow down, I can't understand you." I said.

His mouth simply formed one word, "WHY?"

I tried my best to explain where they would be taking him. I tried to explain how the graft had not sealed right and that it needed to be repaired. I told him that it was possible that a couple of stitches through the back of his mouth might take care of it. By the time I was finished, Steve was crying. I held on to him and told him that I was going to stay with him until it was time for him to go.

Questions: Where are they suturing?   **G R A F T ON DURA (COVER TO BRAIN)**

How are they doing it?   **THROUGH THE MOUTH OR ELSE REOPEN**
What are the risks?   **THE SAME AS BEFORE**
How long will it take?   **???**
Another cisternogram and if so when?   **IN ABOUT TEN TO TWELVE DAYS.**

Steve is very alert and aware of surgery today. Asking

questions. They will attempt to correct leak by going through the mouth, but if they can't they will have to reopen. They won't know until they start.

Being done at Mass. Eye and Ear.

Spoke to Dr. Gress this afternoon; he reassured me that everything would be all right. Minor compared to what he has already been through.

Surgery begins at 6 o'clock tonight.

It seemed like that day just dragged on forever for Steve and myself. They put him on what is called the Operating Room On Call List. Which meant you waited until one became available.

Steve barely slept at all during the day. Each time I felt as though he was drifting off, I would try to slip my hand out of his and redo the restraints. But as soon as I started to leave the room he would wake up.

We "talked" about everything. I explained in more detail to him everything that had happened so far. We would cry together over it. He seemed to understand and accept the fact that there would be a surgery done today. He, just like anybody else, simply wanted it to be over.

Finally at about five o'clock, a nurse came in with a portable oxygen tank and monitor. She placed it on the end of his bed, "He'll be going in about fifteen minutes. You can walk with him over to Mass. Eye and Ear if you want to."

"I don't think so." I said. I looked at Steve. "I think as soon as it's time for you to go that I better leave." My eyes were filled with tears. "If anything happens, if you need me for any reason, I can be back here in ten minutes flat. I think I would be better off waiting this out at my Mom's." I was so tired, not only in a physical sense, but emotionally I was drained.

He nodded his head and reached out for me. I put my arms around his shoulders. We just held onto each other for a few minutes. When I pulled away he just smiled and gave me the thumbs up sign.

"I know everything will be fine. Us Merrow's don't settle for anything less. Remember that." I kissed him, but I could feel the lump starting to get bigger in my throat. If I stayed in that room much longer, I was going to fall apart. I was so scared and I didn't want him to see that. I told him that my Dad was waiting for me downstairs.

"One more kiss good bye and then I have to leave." I said

Once more, I got a thumbs up.

WEDNESDAY NIGHT:

Dr. Ogilvy called at eleven o'clock that night.
It was all done. Steve is just getting back to his room.
They had to REOPEN!
Small graft to help repair the leakage.
It had been taken from the soft pallet in his mouth.
Feels confident that this will do it.
Ten to twelve days to heal
Ten to twelve days to have another cisternogram
Won't keep in ICU that long but not saying how much longer.
More packing.

That night was spent much like the past eighteen nights. Crying myself to sleep wondering how Steve could possibly be feeling.

THURSDAY JUNE 4, 1992

I had called his mother the night before as soon as I had heard from the doctor and explained what he told me. The only ones left to tell were his sisters.

I spoke to his older sister, Linda, and went over everything. She seemed to take it fine but had a lot of questions. I tried my best to answer them for her. The only thing I didn't know was whether or not his face was as swollen as the last time.

Next was his younger sister, Diane, I knew she was at work so I called his mother back to find out how to get in touch with her.

I told Diane everything as well. She was easier to explain things to because I could use the same terms that were used with me. Her medical knowledge was so helpful sometimes.

Then I called my friend, Linda. She started crying on the phone. Her heart was breaking for Steve and for me. She kept telling me that she was sorry she couldn't be here with me. She wanted to be able to do something to help. I wanted to cry. I wished that I could make her understand that she was already doing more for me than anyone could possibly imagine. She had my four children. Knowing that, knowing Linda would take care of them and comfort them when they needed it was the biggest help of all.

A.M. nurse – Cheryl
He is doing fine.
Splint and bandage back on face.
Right eye swollen shut again.
Sleeping all day.

Headache this morning. Had to give him morphine.
Two people from anesthesia were in to see him.
Wanted to test him for a new trachea.
Too sleepy to do it today.
Will try and retest and re-evaluate tomorrow.

According to Cheryl, almost time for a new
ventriculostomy.
Drain needs to be changed to avoid infection.
B.P. looks good.
Had to be put on ventilator for surgery.
Off this morning. Good!!
Nineteen days here.
Steve I need you!!!

Steve has to start coming back to me.
I need him so badly to smile at me again.
To just look up and say it is going to be fine.
Even a thumbs up today would be nice.
Please, dear Lord, give him the strength to fight again!

Another ventriculostomy?   **YES**
What chance is there of him having more leakage?
ALWAYS THAT CHANCE
Does it look like there may need to be a shunt? **N   O   T**
ABSOLUTE

When I asked Dr. Ogilvy these questions, I could tell in his voice that he was holding something back. Not about the chance of there being more leakage, but rather about the shunt. He always told me straight out what he had on his mind. This would be the third drain. I had a feeling deep down inside that the shunt was inevitable.

FRIDAY JUNE 5, 1992

A.M. nurse – Cheryl
Temperature at 102 degrees last night
Up and down all day.
Getting a sponge bath to bring it down.
Physical therapy to start today.

I met his physical therapist today. Her name is Rita. She is a small oriental woman. Extremely nice to both Steve and myself.

She said that her first session with him went very well. He shows extremely good strength in his legs for the amount of time that he has spent in bed. She told me that they gave him a real good work out.

She seems very concerned with the stiffness in his neck. After the surgery his neck was very swollen and he favored his right side. Now, however, he could not move it very well or without pain to the left side. She told me to encourage him to move it, to stay on the left side of the bed. She went so far as to put a sign behind his bed asking everyone else to do the same.

SATURDAY JUNE 6, 1992

I was on my own this morning. My parents had left the night before to go to my grandparents' sixtieth anniversary party. They would be back tomorrow. The phone rang and when I answered it, my sister Debbi was on the other end. She wanted to bring me to the party with her and her girls. She put up a good fight. One day. All she wanted me to do was spend one day away from the hospital. She went on about how happy my grandparents would be to see me. How relieved my parents would be if I went. I finally agreed on the stipulation that she get me back by seven o'clock so that I could at least see Steve before the day ended. She agreed.

The day went well, and she had been right. Both my parents and grandparents were very happy to see me as well as being relieved. I suppose that my being there gave them a sense of ease knowing that Steve must be okay if I was willing to leave his side.

Debbi took me home as promised by seven o'clock and then brought me straight to the hospital. Al was waiting for us in the visitor's room. He had a couple of shopping bags with him. They were filled with canned goods and dry food. People that worked with Steve had donated them to the kids and me. I could not believe it. Al said he knew that I would be here tonight, and didn't want to just leave them. So he had waited for me to show up. He had been there for about an hour. He told me that there were also a lot of baked goods from somebody's bakery coming at the end of the week.

I couldn't believe it. These people were total strangers to

me, but they all loved Steve an awful lot to do something like this.

I stayed with Steve for about an hour. I told him all about the gift of love that we had been given. He was groggy and not very responsive, but I think he knew what I meant. He squeezed my hand tight.

The nurse told me that he had been looking for me all day. I felt so guilty for not being there, but I think spending the day with the family did me a lot of good.

SUNDAY JUNE 7, 1992

Temperature at 101 to 102 degrees all day
Dr. Tatta changed ventricular drain back to the other side.
Should be the last one. Still not definite if things are
pointing to the shunt or not.

Possibly in I.C.U. until after next cisternogram.

Really needs to move his head to left. Real stiff.
Still looking to change to talking trachea tomorrow unless
the fever doesn't go down. If fever doesn't break, it will be
put off.
His Mom showed up to visit him. She surprised me.
She was there when I was ready to leave

Steve was confused off and on during the day. Since the confusion had not really gotten any better, visiting was still limited to me.

I had spoken with Meredith, the social worker, and she felt that the family would be able to handle the confusion a lot better if they would consider sitting and talking with her prior to visiting with him. I had taken her number and given it to the family but as of yet, nobody had asked me to set up an appointment with her.

So, I was very surprised when I was leaving that night, to see his mother sitting in the waiting room. I could not believe it. There she was with her friend Tom. Why couldn't she have asked me about this? Especially where Steve was having a bad day to begin with.

I told her as much and agreed to go back in to talk to the nurses. I explained to his nurse that his mother was there and it would be okay for her to visit. I asked that his nurse be available to her. Could there possibly be one in the room with her? I was concerned about the confusion and that his mother may need some help getting through to him. The nurse agreed with me and I went out to get his mother.

Later that night she called me at my mother's house and told me all about her visit. It had gone well and the nurse had let her stay for about a half an hour. I was happy that she had gone. She really had needed to see him. She really needed to see for herself that her son was doing well. It made me feel good to listen to someone else talk about their visit with him for a change.

MONDAY JUNE 8, 1992

A.M. Nurse – Lisa
Temperature down a little
Changing Catheter, blood showing up in urine

Nothing showed up in urinalysis. Steve probably hurt himself by
pulling on catheter

Temperature in the afternoon at 100.4 degrees

Small amount of blood in ventriculostimy line. Nurse said that it was
probably from yesterday and not to worry.

Went to lunch about one o'clock and when I went back in his room about ten minutes later the dressing was off of his face and his nose was bleeding on the left side.
I got the nurse and asked if he had done it because I knew that it was too soon for the bandage to be off. I found the bandage in his hand. He tried to tell us he didn't do it but we knew better. I found blood all over his hand and on his stomach. I don't know how he could have done it. Both hands were restrained and really tight.
The nurse cleaned him up and thought that the packing may have come out. She called for Dr. Joseph.

Dr. Joseph was there within a half an hour.
Said he would be okay as long as he left it alone.

He wants to delay switching the trachea. That could be why they have not been in to do the test. He is afraid of Steve aspirating again. Feels that one or two more days would be better.

I am starting to sit on Steve's left side in hopes that he will turn his head more that way. It seems to be working.
His hands are non-stop. Trying to pull on all the tubes. Trying to see what is hooked up to him.

With me closer to his free hand, he holds on to me more.

It feels good to have him holding my hand or rub my arm.
Or to see if there are any tears on my face.
Once he even checked to see if I was wearing a bra or not and told me that I had better...Too many doctors around, I guess.

P.M. Nurse – Cheryl
Temp up to 102 degrees
Cheryl says that he is a wild man.
Tossing around
Needed to have some morphine to calm him down.
He is his own worst enemy.

The days I spent with Steve became ones that were nothing but a work out. His hands did not stop. He wanted out of his bed. He wanted to get up out of the chair. He would try to take the IV's out of his arms. While I was trying to pull his hands apart, he would try to work his feet so that they were pulling on the catheters. So I would have to restrain his feet. He was constant movement when he was awake. Although the naps in between were short, they were welcome at times. I was so afraid of leaving him alone and even though he was still considered on the critical list, the nurses really could not stay by his side every moment. At least I knew if I was sitting with him, he could not do anything to damage himself.

He hated the bandages on his nose. He would motion that he only wanted to scratch the top of his nose and as soon as I would let go of his hand he would try to pull the bandage off again. It was frustrating for both of us.

I would try to get him to exercise his arms by either arm wrestling with me or by doing the exercises that the occupational therapist had shown me.

The nursing staff all knew that I had to be there. That Steve would listen to me and more importantly, that I would listen to them. They let me stay in with him as long as I needed or wanted to. For as long as Steve needed me to be there. With one stipulation, that I took a break now and then for lunch and to just get some air. They were all so good to both of us.

He was so dangerous to himself. I would try to explain to him that everything that was connected to him was helping to keep him alive. That everything was extremely necessary. But sometimes it did not make a difference. If he was confused, he just couldn't understand.

As I was getting ready to take a short break, I turned from the bed to gather up my purse. As I turned around, I saw him trying to pull the A-Line out of his arm. The A-line was an IV line fed directly into a main artery.

"Steve!" I yelled at him. "Do you want to die?" I could not believe the words came out of my mouth. "If you do, you are going in the right direction!" I quickly took the restraints and put them on both wrists and tightened them. I knelt on the edge of the bed and grabbed his shoulders. I looked directly into his eyes and asked him again, "Well, do you want to die?"

I saw it in his eyes. Something had hit home. He understood. He seemed to relax. I explained to him that if he had pulled that particular line out of his arm, that he would probably bleed to death. That it was in a main artery allowing the nurses to monitor his blood pressure constantly. He nodded his head to let me know that he understood. Then he started to cry. I can't possibly imagine having to have to try and understand what I was trying to force him to understand. Yet in order for me to help to keep him from hurting himself and the miraculous job the doctors had done, he had to start understanding.

I had tears streaming down my face. "Listen to me! If you don't want to do it for yourself, and you don't want to do it for me," I grabbed the pictures of the kids that I had brought in to him and opened the album to a picture of our baby, Becky. "Then do it for her!" I put the picture up where he could see her. "She is going to need her Daddy!" I put my head down on his shoulder and kept on crying.

Suddenly I felt his chin rubbing against the side of my head. I looked up at him. He had tears in his eyes and his mouth was trying to tell me something. All I could make out was that he was telling me that he loved me and that he did not want to die.

I sat there for about fifteen minutes trying to make him understand that he was getting stronger and that he was almost ready to get out of bed. He had to hang in there. He had to keep a fighting spirit, yet he also had to cooperate with what everybody was trying to do for him.

Doctor Gress met me in the corridor as I was leaving. He put his arm around my shoulder and told me that he had heard a lot of what I said. He told me that he knew how hard it was for me to talk to Steve that way, but that sometimes a patient needed a strong voice. He walked me to the elevator and convinced me that I should go home for the day. I had been through enough. He would tell Steve.

TUESDAY JUNE 9, 1992

A.M. Nurse – Lisa
Temperature down to 99 degrees

Some blood in Steve's mouth in the morning. Dr. Joseph in to look at it. Not coming from nose. Nothing to worry about but a change in the trachea will have to wait a day or two.

Steve looking for food!! Also looking for someone to change his trachea.
His sister Diane came in to visit last night.
Physical therapist in at three o'clock and sat Steve at edge of bed with three of them to help support him.
Put in chair.
Occupational therapist (Ms. Mulligan) spoke to Steve. Has to start doing things for himself.

Steve doesn't want me to go home this weekend. Afraid of something happening while I'm gone.

The blood in Steve's mouth came from the area where they had taken the graft. Dr. Joseph said I shouldn't worry about it. He had cauterized the wound and said it should be all set.

I liked Dr. Joseph. He was humorous, yet at the same time never pulled any punches. He felt though, that it was much too soon to change Steve's trachea to one that would enable him to speak. We would have to wait for a few more days. He said we would have to settle for him writing us little "love notes" in the interim.

After lunch Lisa and I gathered all of Steve's belongings and moved them to what was called an intermediate room. It was a step closer to him leaving I.C.U. Up until now his room was a critical care room. He was right across from the nurse's station with monitors hooked up to him to constantly check all his vital signs. In an intermediate room the monitors would come off, the A-line would finally come out and within a few days he would be transferred to a regular room out of I.C.U. It was a very big step.

The A-line had been in since the first day Steve was at the hospital. It was like a catheter inserted into a main artery in his arm. It was held on with a couple of stitches and was connected to a monitor, which gave a constant read out of his blood pressure. The line was transferred from one arm to the other every other week, but was the one thing Steve constantly tried to pull at. I was so relieved when it finally came out.

When the physical therapist came in at three o'clock, she was accompanied by her assistant. They sat Steve at the edge of his bed with one of them on either side of him. His day nurse joined them and knelt on his bed directly behind him. On the count of three they helped him to stand on his feet. He must have stood there with their support for a solid minute. He was very dizzy, but I felt so good being able to see him on his feet. It wasn't only me who was excited about this accomplishment, either. There were quite a number of nurses at his door cheering and applauding when he stood up. This was a day that we had all worked very hard for.

They sat Steve in a chair for a while before getting him back into bed. Steve looked very upset. I told him how happy I was that he had done so well, but he just shook his head in disgust. His mouth started to go a mile a minute. I got his clipboard and pen and told him to write down what he was trying to say.

His note read, "I didn't GO anywhere! I just stood there!"

So he wanted more! That was terrific. His standing there was enough for me...for now.

That afternoon, before I left, I hung up all of Steve's cards in his new room, and placed all of his stuffed animals in good view.

His "animals" all had very special meanings. There was a small bear that I had bought him the first time I went home to see the kids. He was there to make sure that Steve behaved himself. There was another larger bear. This one came from the kids. Then there was George. George was a small purple dog. I had taken it from Steve's truck the first time I had gone home. George meant a lot to Steve and held a special significance to him as well. Steve had won him in a vending machine. I had tried to lay claim to George, but Steve said it was his dog. That George would sit on his dashboard and would always be there to protect him. Well, George had done his job well. Now George's job was to watch over Steve here.

Steve always held onto George. George went everywhere. To every test. Where eve Steve went, George was with him. H would hold on to him when they had to draw blood. George was the best dog around. Even the nurses respected our attachment to George. They would always make sure that George was in Steve's hand or at least within reach.

I told Steve that this weekend I would be going home again to see the kids. He took the clipboard and wrote to me that he did not want me to go. He said he was all alone and needed me to be there for him. He wrote that he was terrified that something would happen to him and I would not be there to help. I tried to calm him down and told him that everything looked good. I reassured him that if anything did go wrong that I would come right back. I told him that he did not have to worry.

WEDNESDAY JUNE 10, 1992

A.M. nurse – Suzanne
Temperature at 99 degrees
Used a walker to get from bed to chair
Sat in the cardiac chair for forty minutes.
Tried to tell me that he was able to get to the hallway and that he would show me. But I knew better.
Maybe he felt that the walk from the bed to the chair was not that long of a walk.
Pulled the dressings off of the main IV lines. Loosened the IV lines.
Bag off of rectum. One catheter now.
Had a very bad nosebleed. Don't know why. He may have sneezed.
Will be out of I.C.U. in a day or two. Probably gong to the Ellison building on the twelfth floor.
Physical Therapist in to exercise him in the morning.
Change in the trachea delayed again.

I was beginning to wonder if things would ever start to improve. It seemed that each time Steve showed any signs of getting better there would be some set back. The nosebleed was connected to some minor bleeding in his mouth from the area they had taken the graft from. They told me that the bleeding was minor, but it still worried me. Everything worried me. It seemed as though at times Steve was almost ready to give up. I could not let him do that. He was almost there. He was almost ready to start the uphill battle of coming home.

THURSDAY JUNE 11, 1992

His nurse today was Lisa. A young girl whom I had not met until they had moved Steve to his new room. She told me that they were still delaying on changing his trachea. Steve was not feeling that good. I was told it could have been from the bleeding that he had yesterday. It was causing him to have a touch of the diarrhea.

The day was spent much like the ones before. At times I got scared because of Steve's confusion . Once or twice he looked at me and pointed at the door. He was telling me to leave. He didn't want me to be there.

The therapist came in at about one o'clock and got Steve out of the bed. He used the walker and managed to get from the bed to a commode chair without too much of assistance. It made both the therapist and myself very excited. As usual, however, Steve didn't think it was enough. He wanted to get up and just fly. He was not about to settle for a couple of steps. He would not be satisfied until he was ready to run the marathon.

By the time I reached my parents house that night, I was just about dead on my feet. I got about as far as the sofa and simply collapsed. I was totally exhausted. The day itself was not tiring as much as it was stressful. The entire thing was catching up with me and I was about at the end of my energy supply.

My mother ran me a bath and I soaked for about as long as I could stand it. My mind kept going over everything. I was heading home for the weekend and I knew that Steve didn't want me to leave. I would have to talk to him again tomorrow and try to make him understand. I had to go home and spend some time with the kids. They needed to be able to see me and for me to reassure them that Steve was okay. I would only be gone for a day and a half.

FRIDAY JUNE 12, 1992

Graft in mouth bleeding – a lot.
Dr Joseph called – had to cauterize the graft again
Stable
Swallowed a lot of blood
Vomited through trachea
Was told it was not as bad as it looked.

I got to the hospital and buzzed the intercom to be allowed in to see Steve. I was met at the door by his nurse. She said that she wanted to explain to me what had happened to Steve so that I would not panic. Too late. I was already in a state of panic. She said that he had vomited a lot of blood and that it looked really bad. She was in the middle of cleaning him up when I had asked to come in to see him. She was still trying to explain to me what happened but I was pushing by her and going into his room. What met my eyes was beyond words.

He was awake but looked terrified. There was blood everywhere. It was covering the dressing to his trachea and was still on his neck and chest. His pillow was blood soaked as was his sheet. It looked like someone has slashed open a main artery.

I could feel the nurse behind me. "What the hell happened to him?" My voice came out as a whisper and I could feel the room start to spin.

"He had a lot of bleeding from his mouth during the night and swallowed it. Blood in the stomach causes extreme nausea and diarrhea. He vomited it, but a lot of it came out of his trachea tube." She went on to tell me that the doctor had been notified and was on his way over to look at the wound. When she told me that it looked bad, however, what she had meant was that it looked a lot worse that it really was.

I went to the side of his bed. "Are you okay?" I asked him.

He looked at me and nodded his head. He motioned for the pad of paper. When I gave it to him he wrote: "I fucked up. It's all my fault."

I couldn't believe it. How could he possibly blame himself! I looked at the nurse. She assured him that there was no possible way of him doing this on his own. She looked at me and told me that she would have the doctor reassure him when he arrived. She also told me that she thought I should get some air and let her finish cleaning him. I told Steve that I would be right back, and walked down the hall to the lounge. The scene in his room was very overwhelming and I needed to compose myself. Once I had I went back to the room and helped the nurse clean Steve and his bedding.

Later that afternoon, a nurse from the Ellison Building (the building they would be transferring Steve to) came in to introduce himself to Steve and myself. His name was Paul. I thought it was so nice of him to do that. He told me that they were going to move Steve to the Ellison no later than Monday. I asked him if they could wait until Monday because I was not going to be there over the weekend. He said in all probability the move would be done tomorrow.

I looked at Steve. I knew what he was thinking. I told him that it would be okay. I gave him a kiss and told him that I would be right back.

I went to the nurses station and found his nurse. "Is he going to be okay?" I asked.

Barbara nodded her head, "Dr. Joseph was in and cauterized the wound again. He may vomit again and he will definitely have the diarrhea for a few days."

Should I change my plans for the weekend?" I asked her. "I was planning on going home to be with the kids."

She shook her head. "No. He will be fine. If it will make your decision any easier, why don't you ask him?"

When I went back into Steve's room and asked him, he wrote down that he would really like me to stay and not go but he knew that the kids were looking forward to seeing me. I told him that I would be in touch with the nurses during the day and that if anything at all should happen, I would be back in a flash.

This time leaving Steve was hard. Even though the doctors and the nurses told me that the bleeding was under control, they still had to give him two units of blood to replace what he had lost. Between that and him probably being moved tomorrow to a new location, it was hard to leave the hospital knowing that he had all of this happening.

Before I left that night, I spoke to his nurse and made sure that she knew where I would be and how to get a hold of me. I asked her to make sure that if they moved him tomorrow to be sure that George didn't get lost and that all of his cards were moved with him.

As I lay in bed that night, I thought about all of the people who had helped both Steve and myself get through the past month. Not only Dr. Ogilvy and his team, but the nursing staff as well. They had all kept my husband alive. They had constantly watched and cared for him. All of them had always been there for me when I needed something.

His primary nurse Cheryl knew how badly I needed to be able to be close to Steve. She had taken great pains to explain things to me. It was so heartwarming to watch her get excited when Steve crossed a hurdle or made steps towards his recovery. As a nurse, she was excellent. As a person, I will always remember how caring and warm she was.

Then there was Barbara. She must have been tops in her class. She always seemed to know when I needed a shoulder. She became not only Steve's nurse, but my friend. When I had decisions that needed to be made, and she knew I was having difficulty making them, she would help me to see what was best not only for Steve, but for myself and the family as well.

Meredith, the social worker assigned to our case, was also a God-send. She would sit and listen to my endless babbling. She always seemed to go out of her way to get answers for me.

The nursing staff as a whole, although I can not remember all of their names, went above and beyond what I could have ever imagined. Their patience with me and their willingness to help me as the patient's wife, deserves recognition.

The one nurse who will always be special to me, is Dede Buckley. When ever things looked really bad, she seemed to be there for me. She took time out of her day to get me answers or to simply just sit and talk. She was truly our Florence Nightingale.

Dr. Gress, although not directly assigned to Steve's case, was the Chief of Neuro-I.C.U. He was another one who would go out of his way to "check up" on me. He would answer questions for me. A credit to his profession.

Everyone involved with Steve's stay in the I.C.U. are the best professionals in the medical world that I have ever seen. I will always remember them.

I wanted to let them know in a special way how I felt about them. The only way I knew of was in my writing. So that afternoon before I left, I wrote a poem and gave it to them as I was leaving.

Through our darkest hours
You cared for him
Nurturing, caring
Easing his pain.
Hour after hour
And day after day.
You would take care of him
While I'd sit and pray.
With the worst behind us
And a long road yet to tread
Without all of you,
That road would not be ahead.

So to the doctors and nurses
And secretaries too
There is nothing more for me to say
Than a very humble
Thank you

SATURDAY JUNE 13, 1992

Home with the kids.
Will be going back tomorrow
Called the hospital – nurses said he had a good night.
He was moved to the Ellison building.
Nurse said in the afternoon that he was sitting up, looking
out of the window.

I must have called the hospital four or five times that day. I tried to relax and enjoy my time with the kids. His sister Linda was throwing a birthday party for her two older children tomorrow. The kids would be able to be with the family and have a fun day. We wrapped gifts and had another pizza party that night.

Our friend Marybeth came by to visit and we played cards. As we talked, she wanted to know if I needed help with anything. I explained that the only thing I really needed was somebody that would be able to watch the kids on the weekends that I should not be able to make it home. Linda needed a break and I really didn't have anybody else to do it. She told me "No problem." What really struck my heart was that she meant it. I told her that I would keep her in mind.

The night was long and lonely. I checked in with the nurses to see how Steve was doing only to get the same reply that I had gotten all day. He was doing fine. He was having a good night. I couldn't make the night pass fast enough.

SUNDAY JUNE 14, 1992

I don't think I slept for more than an hour or two that night. I kept remembering how intent Steve was about me not coming home. I felt as though I had deserted him. It was so unnerving.

I went out to the kitchen and had some juice. I picked up the phone and dialed the number to the hospital. As it was ringing, I looked at the clock. Two-thirty in the morning. I hung up the phone. They would probably think I was nuts. I felt as though I was nuts.

Besides, if anything was wrong, they would call me. Right?

I tried to convince myself of one thing, I had to be a mother as well as a wife. My kids were being pulled apart by this and they needed me as much if not more than Steve did.

I went back to bed and probably got about an hour more of sleep before I started to hear Becky stirring in the other room. I went out to the kitchen and started a pot of coffee. I was going to need a lot of caffeine to get through the day.

It seemed as though everything set me off. I was yelling at the kids for no apparent reason. They simply looked at me as though I had two heads. They didn't know what was wrong with me.

This morning I woke up feeling uneasy and nervous.
Maybe it's the kids
Maybe I just don't want to leave the kids again.
Maybe this whole thing is getting to me.

I called the hospital
Got the same response as yesterday

He had a good night.
No changes

I didn't know what was wrong with me. I was snapping at the kids, and was on edge all morning. I got the little ones dressed and ready for the party. I had told my sister-in-law that I would bring the kids at one o'clock. I would try and get there early so that I could spend time with my niece and nephew but then I would have to be on my way by about two thirty.

I got dressed in my white summer dress and headed over to her house at one o'clock. I just could not shake the nervous feeling that I had. I decided that it must be the fact that I had to leave the kids at Linda's house. Again, I must be feeling guilty about not being with them.

I talked to my sister-in-law about it and she told me not to worry about the kids. They would be fine until my girl friend Linda got back to get them. It didn't seem to help though.

As I was pulling away from her house and waving good-bye to them, I started to cry. I could not understand why I was crying though. The kids were fine and they were going to have a fun filled day. I was on my way back to the hospital and I would be with Steve in about an hour.

When I reached my house Al was waiting for me. He would be driving me back to Boston. I wiped my eyes as I got out of the car. I only hoped that he wouldn't notice that I had been crying. I think if he asked me what was wrong, I would have started crying all over again. I smiled and thanked him for helping me as I got in the car. I told him that my parents would meet me at the hospital in a while and would be able to take me back to their house. I asked him if he could wait with me until they got there. He said he would and we started the ride back to Boston. I just sat there quietly watching the cars. I couldn't shake the uneasy feeling I had.

Got to the hospital about four o'clock
Steve is really confused
Something is wrong

When I got to the hospital and found Steve's new room in the Ellison Building it was about four o'clock. He was sound asleep and looked very content. As always. I looked at the chart by his bedside to see what his vital signs were. They looked good although his blood pressure and pulse were a little high. Then I noted the bag that was connected to the drain on his head. There was a piece of tape on it with the time noted. That was odd. I had never noticed them doing that before. The time noted was seven o'clock that morning. It appeared that there had not been anything added to the bag since that time.

I looked at the area where the dressing was for the drain. To me, it appeared to be swollen. I could have been wrong. I went out to the nurses station to find out who his nurse was. I was introduced to Greg and asked him to come into Steve's room. I pointed out to him what I thought was swelling and Greg agreed with me.

Greg left the room saying that he would see if the doctor who was on duty would come in and look at Steve. While he was gone Steve woke up.

His mouth was moving. He was trying to ask me where I had been. I didn't understand. He knew that I had gone home. At that moment, Al walked into his room.

"Hey, big guy!" Al said, "How are you doing?"

I looked at Al and then back at Steve. "Steve, do you know where you are?"

Steve nodded his head. He said he was in the hospital. I asked him where. His mouth moved forming the words Hampton Harbor.

I was getting scared. Something was definitely wrong. I looked at Al and told him I would be right back. I wanted to talk to the nurse.

Greg was still at the nurses station. I went over to him and asked him if he had found the doctor yet.

"Is something else wrong, Mrs. Merrow?" he asked.

"Yes. He seems really confused. He doesn't remember that I had gone home for the weekend. He wants to know where

I've been. He also thinks he is in Hampton." My hands were shaking.

"I've just gotten off the phone with the doctor. He has asked that we get a CT-scan done."

I was right. Something was wrong. CT-scans were never done on weekends, unless it was an emergency.

The nurse looked at me and said, "Don' panic. He was due for a follow up CT-scan anyway. Maybe this is it." Gregg told me that he would be brought down to radiology and that the test would be done within the hour.

I went back into his room. Al was talking to him about the store and their friends. Al could tell by the look on my face that I was upset.

I told Steve that in about an hour or so he was going to be going downstairs for a CT-scan. He looked confused and scared. I told him it was just a follow up and that I would be here when it was over. I held his hand and bent down to give him a kiss. When I looked up my parents were walking into the room.

I stayed while they had their visit. Then I walked down to the lounge area with my parents and Al. I told my parents about the test he was having. My mother looked scared. I told her not to worry. That it was just routine.

"It will only take about an hour, and I promised Steve that I would be here when he came back upstairs. Is that okay?" I knew that my father would not want to fight Sunday night traffic going back home, but I just couldn't leave.

"Don't worry about it Laura." He said, "We will stay and take you back afterwards." My Dad turned to Al, "If you want to take off, we'll be able to stay with Laura until Steve gets back."

Al just shook his head. "No, that's okay. I think I'll stay. I'll wait until she finds out what they see. I just want to be sure that everything is going to be okay." Al knew that it was more than just a routine test being done. He knew that I was scared.

We waited until they had taken Steve down to radiology and then my Mom and I went to Brigham's for a cup of coffee. We weren't there long before my Dad and Al walked in. We sat and drank our coffee and tried to pass the time with idle talk.

When I knew that it was almost time for the test to be over we all walked back. As we walked into the hospital, and entered the hallway that took us to the elevator bay, I could hear someone being paged. "....please return to Ellison twelve. Mrs. Steven Merrow....please return to Ellison twelve immediately..." My heart nearly stopped. The page was repeated as I stood completely still and numb. It wasn't until I heard it for the third time that I moved. Then I ran. I bolted for the elevators. Something had happened. Something had been found and I was not there like I had promised Steve I would be. I pushed past the people in the corridor and ran to the elevators. By the time the elevator doors opened, my parents and Al had caught up to me. We all went upstairs in the elevator. Once the doors opened, I bolted for the nurses station.

"Here she is!" A nurse was pointing at me and speaking to a doctor dressed in hospital greens.

"Mrs. Merrow?" He introduced himself as a Dr. Pacsaban.

"What's wrong? Has something happened to my husband?"

"Mrs. Merrow calm down. He has just been brought up from radiology and is being settled. The nurse tells me that you were concerned about some confusion in your husband. These are subtle changes that cannot be seen by someone who is not familiar with him." He went on to explain why the hospital staff could not detect these 'subtle' instances of confusion. My concerns were justified.

He spoke very quickly and seemed to want to get directly to the point. "We have noticed that the ventricular drain has not been putting out an awful lot of fluid. Between that and the confusion you noted led us to want to get the CT-scan done."

I was terrified. Something was happening and Steve was in danger yet again. The doctor was talking about the results of the scan. "We saw a clog at the base of the drain. The swelling you saw is the beginning of hydrocephalus."

I knew what that was. Dr. Ogilvy had explained that to me in the beginning. Swelling of the brain. The doctor continued.

"There is some swelling of the brain starting and we will need to place the shunt in tonight."

"I know what the shunt is, Dr. Ogilvy explained that to me when Steve was brought in. I had a feeling that it was going to be necessary. This has to be done tonight?"

"Yes. We are going to be taking him down very soon. We just have to find out which operating room is available. As soon as I have it ready, I will need you to sign a consent form."

"Does Steve know about any of this?" I asked.

"Not yet. We had to discuss it with you first. Do you want me to go in with you to tell him? Or would you like me to tell him for you?"

"No. I'll tell him. It will be easier on him if it comes from me." I looked at the clock. It was about five-thirty. "When will he be going?"

"As soon as possible." The doctor turned and went back to the desk to prepare a consent form for the surgery.

I turned around to my parents. My mother came to me and put her arm around my shoulders. "Everything is going to be all right, Laura." She gave me a hug and then said, "Why don't you go in to him and we will be back in a few minutes." I nodded my head. She was right. I had to be alone with Steve for a few minutes. He needed to hear this from me, and I needed to tell him before they started prepping him to be moved.

I walked into his room. He was asleep again. The doctor had called that being lethargic. Sleepy.

I sat on the edge of his bed and called his name. "Wake up sweetheart. Come on Steve, please, wake up for me."

His eyes opened. He looked at me and his mouth was moving asking me what was wrong. Why did I wake him up?

I told him that he was having a problem and that he needed to have an operation. I told him that they were going to be replacing the drain on his head. I didn't want him to be scared, but I also wanted to let him know what was happening.

I explained to him about the shunt, and it would be placed inside his head and that it would do the same thing that the drain did now. That it would only take a few hours and that he would be brought back to the same room when it was over.

A woman that I had not met before came in. She introduced herself as Betsy. She was the night nurse. She wanted to know if I was okay. I told her not to worry about me. I asked her if I would be able to stay at the hospital and wait until the surgery was over.

She told me that whatever I wanted to do was okay. Steve started to ask her something and she stopped him. "Listen you, you are going to be fine. We are going to take good care of you. Right now I want to be sure that your wife is okay."

I told her that I was going to get some air and asked if he would still be here when I got back. She told me that it would be about fifteen minutes before he left. That I should get some air and pull myself together.

I went down to the lounge and Al was still sitting there. He said that my parents were out in the courtyard having a cigarette. We went outside and I updated them on what was going on.

My mother looked at me and told me that I should come back to the house for a while. My father said he would bring me back to the hospital later on if that was what I wanted to do.

I shook my head. I didn't want to leave. Al told them that he would stay with me. I took a puff off of my father's cigarette and they should decide what they wanted to do and for someone to let me know because I was not leaving. If I had to I would take a cab back to the house. But that I wasn't leaving Steve until he was back from surgery.

I went back upstairs. I hadn't been in with Steve for more than a minute or two before they were at the door to take him.

While they were getting him prepared to be transferred, I went back out to talk to Dr. Pacsaban. He quickly went over the risks to the operation and had me sign a consent form. There were a lot of questions that I had, but I knew that there was not enough time to ask them.

CT-scan showed a clog in the drain

Will have to do surgery – shunt permanent
Dr. Pacsaban and Dr. Barker to do surgery tonight.
Long term risks: *Shunt malfunctioning*
(then he would need to have a new one)
Infection – watch fevers

As they wheeled Steve down to the elevators, I started to cry again. Betsy came over to me and held on to me. She tried to comfort me, but her efforts were to no avail.

I stopped crying, but I was very shaky. She had another nurse get me a cool cloth. I put up a fuss, but she was right and I knew it. I felt faint and needed to be cared for.

"You know it is okay for you to fall apart. It is very healthy. Your husband is in good hands. You have to realize that."

I knew that she was right. It didn't matter though. Al came over to me and guided me down to the elevators and then out to the courtyard. My parents had headed home and Al was enlisted to try and convince me to follow them. Even if only for an hour or two. They thought that I should get away from the hospital and relax a little. I agreed with Al on the condition that within an hour or two somebody would get me back to the hospital. I had promised Steve that I would be there when he woke up. That I would stay at the hospital while he was being operated on. He had even handed me his dog George. I had to hold on to George for him. He told me that George could take care of me while he was in the operating room. That he wanted me to take care of George as well.

I went back upstairs to the nurses station and told Betsy that I was going to my parent's house for a couple of hours and that I would be back. She told me to relax. That there would be no problem with me coming back in.

Once back at the house, I made a call to my sister-in-law to let her know what was happening. Before I had a chance to explain anything that was happening, she was going on about how my girlfriend had not made it to pick up the kids yet. That nobody knew where she was, other than on her way back from Maine. She had been expected hours ago. The children were all tired and she said at this point she was about to find places for them to fall asleep.

I stopped her in mid-sentence and told her about the surgery. I told her that I knew how crazy it was there but I didn't know what to tell her other than to say I was sorry about the mix-up.

She apologized. She had no idea that I had called with bad news. She didn't mean to dump more problems or worries on me.

"Linda," I started to say to his sister, "Can you call your mother and fill her in on what is going on?"

"Ma's here with me" she said.

We talked for a few minutes and I told her that I would call her as soon as everything was over.

My mother in the meantime was fixing me something to eat. I didn't have the heart to tell her that I was not at all hungry. I sat at the table and tried my best to eat, but it was no use. My stomach was in knots.

After about two hours, I couldn't take it any longer. Al drove me back to the hospital and we sat in the lounge. I clung to George for dear life.

Al fell asleep after a while and I paced. At about midnight I tried to call Linda Grant to see if she was back from Maine yet. She answered the phone and went right into an explanation of what had happened. I interrupted her and told her that I was at the hospital and that Steve was being operated on again.

She started to cry. We talked for a while longer and I went back into the lounge. I sat holding onto George for what seemed like an eternity. I must have dozed for about five minutes, only to be woken up by a nurse. "Mrs. Merrow?"

I jumped up. She told me that Dr. Barker was on the phone and wanted to speak to me. I ran down the hall and grabbed the phone.

He told me that Steve was in recovery and that the surgery was over. Everything went smoothly. I told him that I would be waiting in the lounge until Steve came upstairs in case he needed me.

Al was awake when I went back in. I told him to go home and that I would take a cab back to my parent's house. He said he had waited this long and that he would wait until Steve had come back upstairs and then take me back home.

I called Steve's sister and my girl-friend to let them know it was over. When I got off the phone, Al took me downstairs to the vending machines for a cup of coffee. We went outside to smoke a cigarette. Al tried to convince me that everything would be fine. But I knew that until I saw Steve, my thoughts could not be changed. I needed to see him back in his room. I needed to have this over.

Surgery went smoothly
Steve awake
Incision on stomach painful
Went home at about 2 AM

When I went to Steve's room, he was wide awake, which really surprised me. I stood by his bed and he reached out for my hand. He had bandages on his head and neck. There was also a bandage on his stomach. They had shaved half of the hair off of his head.

I stayed with him for about a half-an-hour. Betsy came in and gave him a shot of morphine. When I knew that he was about to drift off to sleep, I told him that I was going home. I gave him a kiss and said good night. Before I left I put George by his pillow and told Betsy not to let him fall on the floor. At first she thought I meant Steve, then she laughed when I explained that I meant the dog. I told her about George and she assured me that George would not leave the bed. I watched as she took a piece of hospital tape and secured George to the guard rail of the bed.

Al brought me back to the house. I had him sleep on the couch. My Dad also insisted that he stay. It was two-thirty and there was no way either one of us wanted Al going all the way back to Derry.

I lay in bed for a long time praying to God to end this

nightmare. Steve had been through enough. How much more could he take? If God was testing us, Steve and I had both passed.

MONDAY JUNE 15, 1992

Temperature down – Blood pressure fine
A.M. nurse – Karen / Leann
Sleepy from the surgery
Slightly confused in the morning but much
Better in the afternoon.

Surgery last night explained better:
SHUNT: draining fluid that is not being absorbed by
the brain. It is being redirected to the stomach through a tube
which starts in the ventricles of the brain. The tube
runs down a vein in his neck and then goes down into
his stomach.

Hair shaved on most of his head. Two small bandages on
head. One on neck and one on stomach.
Spoke to a nurse on what to expect from drain. She
Explained more about the surgery.
Dr. Ogilvy called and said that Steve looks good. Everything
Neurologically looks fine.
The cisternogram is planned for either Wednesday or
Thursday.
The packing will come out on that day.
I need to talk to a social worker about a rehab.

This whole thing seems so unreal.
I feel so helpless and vulnerable. I sit and watch the doctors
and Nurses and want so badly to wake up and have this
whole nightmare come to an end
You wrote to me that you feel sad and lonely without me and

the kids. I wish I could spend every moment with you, but I know that I can't
I feel so guilty when I have to leave the hospital when I'm tired because I know
That you are going through so much. The nurses look at me and want help. But until you are back home, I won't be better.

Lump on top of Steve's head????
Spoke to Dr. Pacsaban and he told me that it was the shunt. That Steve's hair would grow back over it.

Steve slept for a good part of the day. The nurses came in off and on to check on him. The visiting regulations were different here. Anyone could see him. The hours were from one o'clock to eight o'clock at night. I had made arrangements to be able to come in between eleven and twelve. As long as the nurses had finished with Steve in the morning and I didn't get in their way.

His primary nurse was Karen. A small girl but very good at what she does. She was accompanied by another girl by the name of Leanne. She was a graduate nurse and very nervous. She reminded me a lot of my sister-in-law Diane. I told Leanne that my sister-in-law had also just graduated from nursing school.

I was very tired today. Last night had been extremely tiring and stressful. I sat in the chair next to his bed trying my best not to fall asleep. From time to time I would try and ask Steve how he felt. Other than a lot of pain from the incision on his stomach, he seemed to be doing fine.

He was very confused though. I would have thought that the surgery would correct that but the doctors and the nurses told me that it would take some time.

I hung up all of Steve's cards and pictures from the kids. I found an envelope full of drawings from Jimmy's classmates. All of them had little get well messages on them. I picked out about ten of the best and hung them up as well. I would show some of them to Steve and he would nod his head in approval.

He asked for the clipboard in order to write something to me. He wrote that he did not understand why Dawn's class had not sent pictures. It said that she had promised. I felt my heart drop. Dawn wasn't in school yet. I took the clipboard from him and explained to him that Dawn was drawing him pictures but that she hadn't finished them yet. I was so afraid of getting him upset.

It scared me so much when he got confused. I was so afraid that if he got upset, something would happen. I also had this fear that the confusion would never go away.

He was told that he had to lie flat on his back for the day. Each day they would raise the bed a little more. By doing this his brain would get used to the shunt. It would take about four to five days before they would sit him up and consider getting him back out of bed.

TUESDAY JUNE 16, 1992

When I got to the hospital this morning Karen told me that Steve had been vomiting again. The wound in his mouth was bleeding again and he had swallowed more blood.

I looked at Steve, he was as white as a ghost. Karen told me that she had notified Dr. Joseph and that he was on his way over.

As I sat and tried to talk to Steve, he suddenly got very agitated. He was pointing into the corner of the room and his mouth was trying to form words. I handed the clipboard to him and he was writing very quickly. He was very upset about something and still pointing at something in the corner of the room. When I looked at the clipboard, I really could not make out what it said. He grabbed the pen and in big bold letters wrote that the door of the truck was open. Someone had to shut the door.

I got scared. Karen tried to calm him down. I didn't know what to do or to say. "Steve there is not a truck there. What do you think you see?" I looked at Karen. She was as baffled as I was. "Honey, where are you? Tell me where you are!"

He wouldn't answer.

"Steve," I said. "You are in the hospital, remember?" I sat down on the edge of the bed and looked in his eyes. "Do you remember which hospital you are in?"

He wouldn't answer me. He looked angry as ever and just turned from me and stared out of the window.

Karen pulled me aside and told me it was not uncommon for a patient to have a couple of hallucinations after surgery. To me it didn't matter what she said. The confusion and the hallucinations were scary. I just did not know how to handle them anymore. I was so frightened, and so overwhelmed.

Dr. Joseph came in moments after that and showed me where the bleeding was coming from. The pallet of Steve's mouth had a lot of bare bone. Once in a while the wound would open and it put out a lot of blood. He quickly cauterized the wound and ordered a couple of more units of blood to be given.

That afternoon the confusion was back again. Steve asked me how the little one was doing. I assumed he meant Becky, our baby.

I was wrong.

He told me that he knew Becky was fine, but was concerned because I never mentioned anything about the little guy. I asked him what he was talking about.

He took the clipboard and wrote down, 'our son'. I asked him if he meant Jimmy.

He got very aggravated and wrote down. "No. Becky's twin. Our son."

I took a deep breath. Here we go again. "Steve, you are wrong." My voice was stern and steady. "Becky has no twin. She was born all alone."

He shook his head and just turned and stared back out the window.

I started to cry and told him I would be back later. I had to take a walk. I needed to get some lunch. I gave him a kiss and ran out of the room.

One of the nurses saw me and came after me. I explained to her that I was scared that something was wrong with Steve. I told her about what had happened. I couldn't stay with her though, I simply had to get away. I had to put space between me and the hell that was becoming too real.

I got out to the courtyard and sat down on the steps. I was so afraid of what I was thinking. It was hard enough to have the life that I knew turned upside down. What if it was worse? What if Steve had some type of brain damage? What if things didn't get better for him? Hearing him insist that he had a son that didn't exist was not the only thing. There were numerous occasions when he told me in his writing that he had brought some kind of a suitcase. Not only did he insist that he had it but he knew what was in it as well! How could any of this be within the 'norm'? How could hallucinations or non-existent people be okay?

I felt so alone again. And again, the tears came streaming down my face.

Roof of mouth bleeding again.
Not as much as last Friday, but he still lost an awful lot
and was bleeding again.

Dr Joseph in to cauterize the wound and showed me where
the bleeding was coming from.

He needed two more units of blood.
Stable otherwise.

Confused. Hallucinating. Thinks Becky has a twin brother.
By the end of the day the twin brother had a name.
Utley.
Incision on stomach sore and the pain runs along the catheter
path.

The time spent at night at my parents' house was getting more and more difficult. Each night after dinner and sometimes even before, the phone basically became attached to my ear. The routine was always the same. Call Linda Grant's and talk to the kids, each one would take a turn on the phone. Then I would talk to Linda for a while. After that it got worse. At least with the kids, the heartache was not being with them. Hearing about their days and wishing it was me spending it with them. It was so hard keeping his family and mine up to date on what was going on.

I didn't mind talking to them. But it was getting so difficult to relive the day's nightmare over and over and over again. Trying to make sure that everybody understood what was going on with Steve. I didn't want to not answer the calls or not let people know what was happening, but I was starting to loose my mind.

My mother was a great help. At times she would answer the phone and try to fill in the person on the other end so that I could have a break.

I hated being afraid. I felt as though it meant that deep down inside I might be loosing hope. When I realized how far Steve had come since the beginning, I would know deep within my heart that he would be all right.

I remembered the night before Steve's first operation when Dr. Ogilvy had explained the surgery and all the possible risks involved. I told him and everyone else that as long as Steve pulled through that surgery, that all the other risks were minimal. I still felt that way. Each day that passed by meant one more day closer to him being home. I had to keep reminding myself that I had to accept each obstacle for what it was worth and not try to read into it.

Tomorrow would bring us new hope. Tomorrow would bring us one day closer to getting Steve home.

WEDNESDAY JUNE 17, 1992

The confusion that Steve was showing began to worry me more and more. I remember it was when they needed to repair the graft on the dura that the doctors told me that confusion was a sign there was a leak. What if that was what was happening now? How in God's name could Steve survive another set back like this?

This was all I could think of on my way into the hospital that morning. It was only three days since they had operated on him and maybe that was the reason, but I wasn't sure. I had to talk to somebody about it. I needed reassurance. I needed answers.

When I arrived at the hospital I stopped short at the end of his bed. He looked so good! They had taken the bandage off of his nose. There was a small amount of discharge but I was sure it was nothing. It just felt so good to see him sitting there without the bandage on his face. It was so good to be able to look at my husband. Steve had been clean shaven again and although I knew he didn't want them to touch his beard, at that moment, being able to see his face, my heart felt a little bit lighter.

They were still were only feeding him through the G-tube. He was craving food so badly. Anything would have appeased him. He would ask me for an ice cream sundae. My heart went out to him but I knew that he wasn't ready for food yet. He needed them to take out the trachea first.

I sat on the edge of his bed and held his hand. "Steve," I started, "Do you know where you are?"

He nodded his head and formed the word 'hospital' with his mouth. I handed him the clipboard and a pen.

"Okay, that's right; you are in a hospital, but write down where the hospital is."

He took the clipboard and wrote down 'Hampton Harbor'. I looked out his window at the view. He could see the Charles River and there were quite a few boats out today. I guess it could make one think of Hampton.

"Honey, you are in Boston," I said. "This is Massachusetts General Hospital in Boston."

He started writing again. This time it said something about the place where the city just finished a new building a couple of years ago. I told him that he was right. As a matter of fact the building he may have been referring to was the one he was in. It was called the Ellison Building and was one of the wings of Mass. General.

I went on to explain the events that had transpired over the past month. When I asked him if he understood, he said he did. I wondered to myself how many times he would have to be told. When would he really start remembering?

The nurse told me that tomorrow they would be doing the other cisternogram. If there was any type of leak or any problem, it would show up there.

I felt secure in knowing that my fears would be relieved tomorrow, but at the same time, I was heartsick knowing what he would have to go through during that test.

Cisternogram on for tomorrow
Bandage off nose. Looks so good!!

Still very confused. Thinks his view is of Hampton Harbor
Now thinks that "Utley" is our ten month old son.

Confusion worries me that there is leakage around the graft

Wants out of bed and food!
A lot of air in stomach. Stomach really sore.

Mom M. in to visit.

At four o'clock I left Steve's room and went outside to the corner to wait for my father. He was just pulling up and I got in the car.

"How is Steve today?" he asked.

"Well they took the bandage off of his nose. I guess they are going to be doing the other cisternogram tomorrow." I explained what that test was and what it would show. "Daddy, he is still insisting that we have a son named 'Utley'. He also thinks that he is in Hampton."

My father asked me if I had seen the doctor during the day.

"No, but if there is anything wrong, it will show up in this test that they are doing tomorrow. I'm going to wait and talk to Dr. Ogilvy tomorrow after he has a chance to see the results He'll know more then."

Later that night Steve's mother called me to tell me about her visit with Steve. I had not told her about Steve thinking he had a son.

"Ma, did he ask you anything weird?"

She laughed a little bit, nervously, and then said, "Well he wrote something down, but I didn't understand him. I just did what you told me to do. I changed the subject. Why? Is there something wrong?"

I didn't know how to explain it to her. I didn't want to upset her but I hadn't known that she had planned on seeing him tonight. "Well he gets a little confused about a lot of things. One thing is that he is unsure of how many kids he has."

"What do you mean?" she asked. I could tell by the tone of her voice that she was getting upset.

"He thinks he has a son. Yesterday he thought it was Becky's twin brother and today he claims that this child is ten months old and born before Becky. He even has a name for him. Utley."

"Oh my goodness!" she sounded scared. "Why do you suppose he thinks that? Do you think he is remembering the baby you lost?"

We had lost a baby before Becky was born. I had miscarried

in my fifth month. Both of us took it really hard. So hard, in fact, that it led us to make the decision of having my tubes tied. We found out after the surgery that I was three days pregnant with Becky when they tied my tubes. She was our miracle baby.

"Well I thought about that, but I'm just not sure," I told her that he was scheduled to have a cisternogram done tomorrow. I also told her that I was concerned that his confusion could be connected to a leak like he had before.

She didn't seem to be taking it well. I had to prepare her though. If the test did show a leak, I felt that she had to be ready.

"Would that mean that they would have to operate on him again?" she asked. "Oh my gosh, how could he take another one?"

I tried to calm her down, but I had been asking myself the same types of questions. I told her that we weren't sure what was going on. It was quite possible that there was nothing wrong. Hopefully they would not see any problems tomorrow.

I stayed on the phone with her and tried to be sure she understood. The test was not being done because of the confusion, but simply as a follow up test because of the last time there was a leak. If the doctors were concerned they would surely speed it up. Right now, however, he was confused. The nurses had told me that the doctors were watching him and we would have the answers we needed tomorrow.

Everyone called that night. Al, Linda Grant and Steve's sisters. Friends I worked with. Al told me that he would be going to the hospital tomorrow to see Steve. I explained what was going on. Al said that he would get there before the test so he would have a chance to visit Steve. He said that it was his day off, so if I wanted some company while Steve was going through the cisternogram, he would stay until I got the results. He seemed just as scared as I was so I told him if he was sure he didn't have anything else to do that I could use the company.

Needless to say, that night I didn't get much sleep. I kept thinking of Steve and wishing that this nightmare was over for him. The more he had to go through it seemed to me that things only got worse.

THURSDAY JUNE 18, 1992

A woman by the name of Paige came by to see Steve today. She is from occupational therapy. She sat with him for about an hour asking him routine questions. She told me that he was still extremely disoriented about where he was. Sometimes he told her Hampton, and then sometimes he would say he was in Concord. She emphasized with me that it was a common problem for a patient who has been in the hospital for as long as Steve. Considering the type of surgery he had, that they become disoriented, as she put it, to where they were.

I explained to her about 'Utley' and that Steve still insisted that it was his son. Our son. Paige explained that sometimes a patient would have a dream and it would seem very real and vivid. When they woke up, sometimes it was hard to distinguish between the dream and reality.

I told her that I understood what she was trying to say, but that he was insistent on it. I had tried to ask him if he dreamt it, but he was so adamant about it.

Paige told me that if I was that worried about it that she could send in a neuro-psychologist to speak with Steve. I wouldn't agree to it. Not yet anyway. Steve would really freak out if a 'shrink' was sent in. He wouldn't understand. I didn't want to upset him.

Dr. Joseph was in and took the packing out from Steve's nose this morning. This would enable them to do the cisternogram today. It was scheduled for twelve o'clock.

Al came to see Steve about a half an hour before. He stayed in the room for a few minutes and then told me he would be in the lounge. He was trying to give us some time to ourselves.

I hadn't gotten more than two or three sentences said before the nurse came in to tell us that they were ready to take him to radiology.

I gave him a kiss for luck and handed him George. "Squeeze him really tight if you don't like what they are doing. It will be over in a couple of hours." I gave him a kiss and a hug. "I'll be here when you get back upstairs. I promise."

Karen turned to me, "He will be down there for at least an hour or two. This would be a good time to go and get something to eat."

I told her that I would probably be leaving the hospital for about an hour to do just that but that when I got back, I was going to be in the lounge.

I went down to the lounge and Al was waiting. "They are going to take him now. Let's go and get some lunch."

We took a walk up to Brigham's. I was not very good company, though. All I could think about was what the results of the test would show.

When we were done eating, Al thought it would be a good idea for us to take a walk. He said it would do me good. So we walked uptown to Government Center and back again. Al tried so hard to cheer me up. He must have known how worried I was. He tried reminiscing about different times that Sue, Al, Steve and I had spent. He would talk about how funny it was to watch the store managers trying to fill in for Steve. Nothing helped. The time dragged on and all I wanted was to be with Steve. To be holding his hand and telling him that everything was going to be okay.

After a while we went back to the hospital and upstairs to the lounge. I looked at my watch. It was almost two thirty. A couple of minutes later I heard the elevator doors open and saw them wheel Steve past the lounge. Thank God! It was over. I went towards the nurses' station and Karen met me and said that it was going to take about ten minutes or so for them to get him settled.

I went outside with Al and had a cigarette. Then I walked out to the main lobby and bought Steve the Herald while Al went on upstairs. I walked out the main entrance and around the building to the courtyard in an attempt to collect my thoughts and get some fresh air. I sat by myself for a moment looking at all the people either visiting with their loved ones or simply taking their lunch break. It was such an odd feeling seeing people going about their daily routine, while my life was in such upheaval.

When I finally got back upstairs, Al was with Steve in his room along with Rich Chapin. Rich had stopped in to donate blood again and wanted to see Steve.

Both of them left after a while and I was left sitting on Steve's bed. I told him that I would be right back and went out to the nurses' station.

Karen was sitting at the desk. "Karen," I started, "Did they give you a preliminary report on the cisternogram?"

She looked at me and then back at the chart she was reading. "I was just looking for that." She turned to the last entry sheet on Steve's chart. "They really didn't put anything down and the doctor is not up here to read the results."

"Karen," I said, "They did write something down, though, didn't they?"

She looked up at me and said "Well, yes, but it doesn't make any sense. His doctor will understand it."

I asked her to read me what they had put down. Maybe it would give me some clue as to what they saw. I had been listening to so many doctors use so many different terms that maybe I would have some kind of a hint.

"All it says," as she opened the chart back up and turned to the page which held the last entry. "Is that the CSF," she looked back up at me, "That the cerebral spinal fluid,"

"Yes I know what that means, go on." I was so anxious that I almost jumped over the desk to read the chart myself.

"Okay, calm down! It says that the CSF flowed freely from the lumbar and through the basilar artery." She looked back up at me and I could tell by the look on her face that she really didn't know what to say to me.

"It doesn't say whether or not it leaked when it passed over the area that they did the graft on?"

"No, I'm sorry. I read it word for word." She looked as though she would give anything to be able to answer my question. "All I can say is that as soon as his doctor is given the results that I will either send him in to you, or have him call you at your parent's house."

I was so disappointed that we had to wait longer for the information that we both needed. I went back into his room. After a while a nurse named Theresa came in. Change of shifts. I asked her if any of the doctors had been in. She shook her head no.

"Is there any way of finding out the report on the test that he had done today?" I asked.

She said she would see what she could do. A few minutes later she came back and told me the same thing that Karen had.

I apologized to her. I didn't want to sound like a pest but that I was so very anxious to know if there was any type of a leak detected.

She shook her head again and told me that the doctor would be the one to speak to. I looked up at the clock. It was just about four o'clock and my father would be downstairs to pick me up at any minute.

She thought it would be a good idea for me to leave for the day. She said the entire day must have been extremely stressful. "Mrs. Merrow, you are so pale, you look as white as a sheet. I promise to call you if I find out anything and as soon as I see his doctor, I will have him call you."

She took out a pen and wrote her name and the phone number to the nurses' station. "You call me. I don't care what you want to call for. Call me if you haven't heard from the doctor. Call me if you simply need to talk to someone. But for right now, you should go home."

She was right. I was wiped out. I kissed Steve goodbye and headed outside to wait for my Dad. When my father arrived and I told him what my day had been like, he told me to hang in there. When was this going to end? When would things start to look better?

The phone rang after dinner. It was Theresa from the hospital. "Mrs. Merrow?" she asked, "Dr. Ogilvy was just on the phone with me and I explained that you were very anxious to hear the results. Well, I've got only two words for you." She paused then said, "No leak."

I could tell that she was as excited as I was about the results. I thanked her for calling me and asked her to let Steve know. She also told me to feel free to call any time if I needed to talk. She was so helpful. I told my parents and asked my mother to please let anybody who called know the news. I wanted to lie down for a while.

Temperature and blood pressure okay.
Stomach very sore. Cramps.
Al and Rich Chapin in to visit. Rich donated blood again for
Steve.
Changed dressing on G-tube. Still asking for "Utley" and disoriented when it comes to where he is.
Had a math test of sorts and passed. Won't argue when you tell him he's in Boston.

No Leak!!! CT-scan soon
Why the confusion???

Words could not describe how relieved I was when I heard that there was not another leak. The thought of having him need more surgery was more than I could bear. I just didn't know how much more he could take. I didn't know at this point how much more I could take either.

I retreated to my brothers' room and shut door. As I lay down and rested my head on the pillow, I could start to feel the exhaustion overtake me. I drifted off to sleep....

ॐ

I was sitting at the end of a corridor surrounded by a group of nurses. At the other end of the corridor I could see the doors to the I.C.U. where Steve had been. The silence of that corridor was deafening.

Suddenly the doors to the unit opened very slowly. As they opened I could see beyond them to the room at the other end. It was pitch black inside.

Dr. Gress appeared and entered the dark room. A flood of light suddenly engulfed the room. Steve was lying on a bed in the middle of the room. A nurse stood by his bed shaking her head. Dr. Gress turned and walked away.

I screamed to him, "Help him! Please, Doctor, help my husband!" I was screaming so loud it hurt. But he didn't hear me. No one seemed to hear me. I started to run towards the room screaming for them to help him. Dr. Gress was shutting the door to the room, but I could see the nurse inside pulling a sheet over his head.

"NO!!!!!" The door slammed shut.

❧

"Laura?"

I sat up.

"Laura, are you okay? The phone is for you. I think it's Steve's mother."

I looked up, my mother was at the door. It was a dream. No, it was a nightmare.

I shook my head, "Tell her I'll call her later."

My mother left the room and I could hear her making my excuses to my mother-in-law. She returned a moment later with a look of concern. I told her I was fine. I could tell by the look on her face that she was worried about me. I wished I could think of some way to reassure her that I would be fine as soon as this entire ordeal was over.

I wondered though, how long that would be.

I called the hospital as soon as I got out of bed that day. Steve was fine. I could not shake the lingering flashes of the nightmare I had yesterday. I saw my mother off to work and got myself ready to go to the hospital. I looked at the clock, it was only quarter to nine. I didn't care. I had to get in to see him. I gathered my things and went out front to wait for the bus. It pulled up five minutes later.

I found an empty seat and settled in. It took about twenty minutes to get to Central Square. I pulled out my book and attempted to get through a couple of pages.

As the bus pulled up to its next stop an extremely boisterous man boarded shouting some obscenities to the passenger that he bumped into on the way onto the bus. It had been raining out and he was soaking wet and looked as though he may have been drinking.

I took a deep breath and tried to swallow my anxiety as he took the seat directly in front of me. I didn't need this. I could now smell the sour odor of stale liquor coming off of him.

"Some people!" he said turning around to me. "You would think that I went out of my way to bump into him."

My eyes never budged from the page in front of me. I could not acknowledge him. That would only open the doors to a conversation and write an invitation to trouble.

I turned the page in my book. I could feel the other passengers looking on.

"Hey missy, did you see me bump into him?"

He was now perched on the edge of his seat with his arm crossed on the back of it. His voice was loud enough to be heard all over the bus as he went on about his adventures of the night before. His story entailed his mother passing away recently and how he had missed her funeral. He was now on his way to the Cambridge Court House. Then he turned back to me.

"Mind you, I am a very religious kind of a guy. Miss, are you a religious person?" His hand reached for the crosses that hung from Steve's chain around my neck.

I grabbed his wrist before the connection was made. "I wouldn't even think about touching them." Then for the first time, my eyes met his. "Leave me the hell alone." With that I jerked his hand away from.

"I am truly sorry if I offended you in any way, Miss." He said. "I really am." The smell of his breath was turning my stomach. He went on to explain how I must feel. How he knew how dangerous it was for a woman, especially a woman as beautiful as me, to be traveling alone on the buses and subways. Somebody sitting across from me told him to leave me alone.

I looked towards the front of the bus. I could see the bus drivers' reflection in the rear view mirror. His eyes caught mine momentarily, but he quickly looked away. He was an older man and trying his best to pretend not to hear the disturbance coming from behind him.

I turned my attention back to the argument between the man bothering me and the other passenger.

"Why?" he was asking. "Central Square is a dangerous place for a lady to be going all by herself."

"Just leave her alone and be quiet," the other passenger told him.

The man turned back to me. "I think I am going to appoint myself your guardian. You should not be alone in a city like Cambridge."

I looked back up at him. "You don't need to be concerned. I'm on my way to see my guardian. If you were smart, you would just leave me alone."

I'd blown it. I should never have opened my mouth, and I knew it. I should have stayed quiet and maybe he would have left me alone in a minute or two. But now he knew he was bothering me, and it was like a game.

"You know something miss." He started, "I am a very dangerous man. However, I know a lot about Cambridge and I know that you need somebody to protect you. I think that someone should be me. The crazies in Central Square will see you and they will go for you. I only want to protect you."

I lowered my eyes back to my book, hoping against hope that he would simply just disappear. No such luck.

"Especially when you are so good looking. You have a gorgeous face and great looking legs." At that, his hand reached out beyond his seat and started to run up my leg.

I grabbed his hand instantly and wrenched it full force back above his wrist. "I said to leave me the hell alone, and I meant it!!" I released his hand with a jerk and focused my eyes back on my book.

"What's wrong with you Missy? What do you think, that I might rape you or something? Well I could if I want to. I carry a knife in my boot!"

With that comment a gentleman in the back of the bus told him to shut his mouth and to leave the lady alone. My heart was racing a mile a minute. I thought I was going to throw up. The man got up and went to the back of the bus to confront the gentleman who was trying to help me.

I looked out the window, my stop was coming up. I closed my book. The woman across from me told me in a quiet voice to stay in front of her when I left the bus.

As the bus neared Central Square, something happened that totally amazed me. As I stood up to leave the bus, four or five people got out of their seats and practically formed a circle around me as I got off and headed for the subway.

I kept looking over my shoulder for him, but he seemed to have been swallowed up in the crowd. Thank God!

I was at the hospital about fifteen minutes later. As I walked through the front doors and suddenly felt so much safer. Yet I still felt so all alone.

Physical therapy due in today. Rita says it is time to get Steve up and walking.

Hoping to have them test him for different trachea today, but he vomited during the night. So I am not sure that they will.

Vomited twice more – no change to trachea.

They took an x-ray of the stomach – no results yet.

Also, could be a problem with the bowels. An ilius they called it.

Nothing to be 'afraid of' – can either correct itself or be corrected.

Minor compared to everything else

Blood in urine – possible urinary tract infection

Spoke with a woman from the Spaulding Rehabilitation Hospital, very nice woman. Steve will be going there soon. Possibly within a week and a half.

Things should start to get better now.

Steve was up out of bed today. He walked over to the door and back with the walker. Then sat in a chair for an hour or so and we played cards. (We both won a game)

The kids are going to be here on Sunday to see him.

My thought to Steve:

I miss you so much. I got a couple of hugs today. I thought I would melt in your arms. (You made the bus ride of this morning seem less real). You made me feel safe again.

I feel my strength just fade away when I leave the hospital.

Each day it gets a little bit harder to draw the strength back in to face another day.

Steve I love you so much. We will see this through. WE are going to be home soon. One day at a time. One step at a time.

I love you.

SATURDAY JUNE 20, 1992

I was never so relieved to have it be Saturday. That meant that my father would be driving me to Boston. I had told my mother about the episode yesterday. I ended up fine, I told her. I handled it, I told her. She still felt the need to tell my father. He was so upset. I told him, that I had taken an earlier bus than I normally take. The people on the bus later in the morning were for the most part elderly woman who were on their way to the mall or into Cambridge to do their marketing.

The day was busy at the hospital. Steve got up and went into the bathroom with the walker. He didn't even need any help from the nurse or myself. He is finally getting some strength back.

I talked to him about the kids and how they would be in to see him tomorrow. He asked if I would be bringing Utley in. I couldn't hold back the tears.

"Steve, there is no baby!" I was yelling. "There is no Utley! You dreamt it or something, but we do not have a son called Utley!"

Then I got up and ran out of the room.

Second x-ray of stomach showed improvement. Bowel sounds and finally movement.

Steve out of bed – walked to the bathroom with walker and without much assistance.
Confused and it is really starting to scare me. I wish I could shake him and tell him to knock it off.

Still has stomach pains. They aren't as bad.

*The nurses are trying to keep me calm. They know how
much his confusion bothers me.*
*I am afraid of what to say. Afraid to start a conversation
that I cannot finish.*
*I hope tomorrow goes okay. I hope the kids help with his
confusion.*

I need him to come back to me.
All the way back. Soon, I hope.

That night as I lay in bed I thought about the one thing
that I never talked to anyone about. What if he was brain
damaged in some way? What if the confusion never went away?
I keep telling everybody that he will be fine as soon as he able to
communicate with everybody. What if I am wrong? How much
longer is this so called I.C.U. psychosis going to last?

I fell asleep on yet another tear stained pillow. The night
engulfed my fears only to terrify me with its nightmares.

SUNDAY JUNE 21, 1992

FATHER'S DAY...

It only seemed right that the children were brought up to see Steve today. It was Father's Day. I showered and dressed up in a skirt and blouse. I wanted today to be as special a day for him as possible.

I asked Marybeth to prepare the kids as best as she could that morning. I explained to them what to expect and they need not be afraid of anything. They seemed fine.

Marybeth would be bringing the kids to my parents' house at about eleven o'clock. She thought it would be easier if they had a few minutes to visit with me before going to the hospital. As soon as I saw my children I showered them with hugs and kisses. I brought them into the kitchen and sat down with them and went over one more time what they should expect to see. I was more concerned about Dawn. She was at such an impressionable age. They seemed okay though.

We all went together in my car. Marybeth drove. When we got to the hospital, Al was there with Ed Moore, a friend from Grossman's. Marybeth and Al stayed with the kids while I went down to Steve's room to make sure that he was ready for them.

A nurse met me at the nurses' station. She told me that the patient in the bed next to Steve was going to be brought down for some testing and that I should wait for about ten minutes while they got him out of the room. His condition required chemotherapy and his face was very swollen.

I went into Steve and told him that the kids would be in

soon to see him. The nurse told me that I should only bring in two at a time, so I asked him who he wanted me to bring in first. I held my breath and prayed that he would not ask for Utley.

He asked for Dawn and Becky.

I went back down to the lounge and as soon as I saw Steve's roommate being wheeled past I took the two little ones down.

Dawn held my hand as tight as she possibly could. As we approached the bed, I noticed that Steve had fallen asleep. He was still wearing the eye patch. It helped him to focus on the TV better.

When we got close enough for Dawn to be able to see him, her grip tightened even more and she buried her face against my leg. She was crying. I bent down and asked her what was wrong. She said she wanted to go back to the waiting room. I looked at Steve, he was still asleep. I turned and hurried her out before she could wake him.

She told me that the eye patch had scared her. I told here that there was nothing wrong with her Daddy's eye. That it was still there. That the patch only helped him to see the TV. That the eye under the patch got tired real easily.

Marybeth took Dawn and Becky while I went back down to see Steve. He was now awake and looking for the kids. I explained about Dawn and told him that it may be better if he could sit up in the chair. I helped him get out of bed and to the chair. After he was settled, I took his bandana and put it on his head to help hide some of the stitches. Then I removed the eye patch.

I went back to see if I could get Dawn and Becky to come back in to see him. Dawn just shook her head.

"Let Danielle and Jimmy go first." She hopped into a chair and put her head down. I couldn't push her. I knew she was scared and I didn't want her that terrified about her father. I also didn't want her to upset Steve. I picked up Becky and told Jimmy to come with me.

Jimmy went right to Steve. They shook hands. I looked at Becky. Her little blue eyes were fixed on Steve.

"Hi Dada" she whispered.

Steve lifted up his hand and waved. She put her head into my shoulder. "No Mama, go home."

She knew it was her daddy, but she was very apprehensive. I walked a little closer. She only started to cry. I told Steve that I would try to calm her down and bring her back in a minute.

As I headed back to the lounge, I saw Al with his friend Ed. "Al, Jimmy is in there with Steve by himself. Stay in there with them in case Steve needs help."

Al motioned to his friend and they both went right in together.

Marybeth was sitting with Danielle and Dawn. Marybeth looked up at me when I walked in. Becky was still crying and Dawn was still upset. "Marybeth, why don't you take Danielle down to see Steve?" I sat down with Dawn and put Becky on my lap. I told them that their Daddy missed them so much and that they should try to go back in to see him. I told Dawn that I knew she was scared but that all I wanted her to do was to try. He was still her Daddy. He just had a few bandages on and he lost some weight.

"Okay Mommy, I'll try." She hopped down from the chair and took my hand. We headed back down to his room. I let go of Dawn's hand hoping that she would walk over to him. She could not muster up enough strength to fight the fears that she had. I felt so bad for her. There was nothing I could do except hold on to her and reassure her that it was okay.

A nurse came in and took Becky from me to help out. She asked if she could get her a cookie. I nodded and she walked away.

As hard as I tried, Dawn could not look at Steve for more than a second or two. She was so scared. I couldn't blame her. My heart was breaking for Steve. He had so wanted to hold his little girls.

Danielle looked nervous, but she seemed to be handling it fine. She worried me sometimes. I felt that she held her emotions in check. But she did seem fine. As did Jimmy.

The entire visit was rough. When it was time to go, I held Becky in front of Steve and told her that we had to leave.

She lifted her head up from my shoulder long enough to look at Steve and wave her little hand. "Bye-bye Dada". Then she pointed at the door. "Go home now."

Danielle gave Steve a hug and told him to get better soon. Jimmy offered his hand for a handshake and decided instead to hug him. My two oldest missed him so much. He was so much more to them than step-father.

I walked them outside. I wouldn't be going home with them. Marybeth would only let me go as far as the end of the walkway. She told me that they would be fine. She would drop them off at Linda's house and to give me a call later on.

I turned around and started to walk back up to the hospital. Al and his friend were walking towards me. "Lauri, we have to..." Al stopped in mid-sentence and looked at me, "Are you all right?"

"Yeah I'm fine. It's just that I get torn up inside when I can't be with them. Dawn needs her mother, and Danielle and Jimmy and Becky..." I just turned around and started crying.

Al put his arms around me to try and comfort me, but it did little good. The arms I needed were upstairs, and the comfort was back in my own home with my family.

"Al, thanks for coming. I'm sorry, I just can't help it anymore."

"Are you gonna be okay?" he looked at his friend. "We have to get back."

I thanked them both for coming, "I'll be fine. Thanks."

I looked towards the parking garage to see if I could catch a glimpse of the car. I wanted so badly to go home and be the mother to them that they so desperately needed. I knew that I had to stay. Steve needed me more right now. It was good to know that the kids understood that.

I headed back upstairs. As I got to his room and stepped behind his curtain, he was back in his bed. I was dumbfounded. He was sucking on a lollipop.

"Where did you get that?" I couldn't believe my eyes.

He pointed to my purse. I looked inside. My mother must have put a handful of lollipops in my purse for the kids. In my hurry to get the kids out of his room, I had left my purse on his bed. The worst part of all was that he was still not allowed any food or drinks yet.

I couldn't take it away from him. I just didn't have the heart to. He just sat there with a grin on his face. He savored every last drop while I stood guard at the end of his bed.

I stayed and visited with Steve until about six-thirty or so and then went back to my parents' house. I retreated to my brothers' room to put an entry into my log when I realized that I had left it in Steve's room. It was the second of two notebooks, and it only had a few days worth of entries in it. Yet I still worried about his reaction to it if he were to read it.

After a few minutes I decided that it might be okay if he read it. Maybe it would help. For all I knew, he wouldn't even notice it. He knows I've been writing everything down, but maybe he won't see the notebook.

Maybe.

MONDAY JUNE 22, 1992

The day was warm and the routine in the morning was the morning was the same. I was still a little leery of the ride on the bus, but I braved it just the same. The "gentleman" never reappeared after that day, however, I was on my guard just the same.

I wondered whether or not Steve had found the notebook. When I got to the hospital, I went directly to his room. The notebook was lying open on Steve's bed and my answer was on the next blank page. Steve was sound asleep. I picked up the notebook and looked down. Steve had written an entry:

> *Lauri,*
> *I just read the front of this notebook and I can*
> *say that no one has liked what I've gone through.*
> *I'll tell you, you're the most understandable woman*
> *there is on this planet. That is why I love you now*
> *more than before.*
> *Determination.*
> *I want to be in Reh. By Friday. Then I'll be home in a*
> *couple of weeks.*

As I read each word, the tears began to build up in my eyes. I loved this man so much. I wanted to wake him and have him hold me. Instead, I decided to go and get a cup of coffee and pull myself together.

I reached for a pen.

Steve –
I love you.....
I'm here...you're sleeping...be back in a while.

I left the notebook where he could find it with ease and headed downstairs to the cafeteria. I took my coffee out to the courtyard and sat down in the sun. My mind drifted ahead to a time when Steve would be by my side enjoying the sunshine. That day would be here soon.

After a while, I gathered my belongings and headed back up to the twelfth floor of the Ellison building. As I turned the corner towards the nurses' station, I stopped dead in my tracks. Rita, Steve's physical therapist was standing next to a chair. She was with Steve. They must have been about a hundred feet from Steve's room. I could hardly believe my eyes. Rita looked up and motioned for me to join them.

"He is doing tremendous work!" Rita said. "He knew you would be coming back and wanted to surprise you!"

I gave him a kiss. "This is so great! Are you okay?"

He nodded his head to assure me he was fine and motioned for Rita to continue with his walk.

He got about another thirty feet further down the corridor before he turned around for the walk back. He was using the walker but only for a minimum amount of support.

I watched each step. Followed his feet every inch of the way back to his bed. He was exhausted when we finally got him back to his room but exhilarated at the same time. He knew that what he had just done was fantastic.

Rita went over some exercises for him to do in bed and then left. I looked at Steve. Seeing him up and about like that was such a good feeling. It was something that I needed so desperately to feel.

I asked him if reading the notebook had upset him at all. He shook his head and tried to say something. I had him repeat it as I watched his lips. "How are the little ones? Are they all right?"

I nodded. "I talked to them last night on the phone. They are fine."

He motioned for the notebook and a pen.

It has to scare them, with the tubes and machines.
My haircut, scars and stitches.

"I talked to them about it all and told them that you would be back to normal in no time at all." My heart was breaking for him. Yesterday must have been so hard on him.

He was leafing through the pages of my notebook. I looked into his eyes and asked him, "Do you want to talk about it?"

He nodded his head. He tried to ask me what had happened to him. I started at the beginning and again went over the events that led to his surgery. When I was done, he asked for the pen back.

Remember, I was getting headaches all the time?

He understood this time. I nodded my head and explained that there was no way of either of us predicting that the headaches were anything more than stress. At that moment an orderly brought in his roommates' lunch and placed it on the bed tray across the room. Steve was still unable to eat anything. I felt so bad. He picked up the pen again...

Steak and potatoes??
Their having pot roast and I can't have any.
I'll get some.   -

I looked at the clock. It was almost one o'clock. I was starving. He watched as I started to gather my things and wrote

The doctors come in and I don't understand them.

He went on to explain that when I left and doctors came in to examine him that he didn't understand them. He asked me not to be gone too long when I went for lunch. I told him I would be right back. He took the pen again...

If you go downstairs, a paper please.

I smiled and told him that after all he did this morning I would get him anything he wanted. He smiled and asked for steak and potatoes instead. I kissed him and promised to be right back.

Took two walks down the corridor past the nurses station. Looking for anything edible.
Able to wash up in the bathroom. Doesn't want me to leave the room for very long for fear the doctors will come in and he won't understand them. Temperature and blood pressure okay. Tube feeding to start up again today, slowly.
Getting ice chips. Starting to realize a little how lucky he is. Part of me want to hide it all and not tell him anything, but on the other hand I feel he has to know because his life may depend on it and it will definitely change.

MONDAY NIGHT:
It seems like it was only yesterday that you and I were sitting in the kitchen drinking coffee and planning our vacation.

Who would have believed that we would have been faced with all of this?
I hope when this is all over and you start comprehending what has happened you'll feel that I did things the way you would have wanted me to.

I feel at times that I am not doing things right or that I am not making the right decisions.

I know that medically what has gone on has had to be

in order to keep you alive. The Doctor says I ask a lot of GOOD questions and that I ask all of the right questions. Well, I have to. They have your life in their hands and I want to be sure I understand what is happening for me to be able to explain it to you.

TUESDAY JUNE 23, 1992

On the tube feed again – finally. They started him at
80 mg. per hour. They will increase up to 120 mg per hour.

Consultation done on trachea. They want to change to a tube
feed that has blue dye in it.

Possibly, hopefully, they will change the trachea tomorrow.
Occupational therapist in this morning. He is doing fine.
She checked his motor skills.

They stopped giving him ice chips. I talked to Dr. Leng.
Why stop the ice chips? What problems have they caused?

Steve got very upset when they stopped the ice chips. He couldn't
understand why. Neither could I but I had to abide with the
doctors decisions. They knew best. Right? He wanted me to
sneak him in some ice. When I wouldn't do that he wanted me
to give him a lollipop and watch for the nurses. When I refused
him on that he got angry at me and told me to leave the room. I
tried to make him understand, but it was no use. He closed his
eyes and drifted off to sleep.

I went out to the courtyard and found a corner. I sat down
and cried. I wished that he would understand. I took out my
notebook and wrote Steve a note. I didn't know if or when I
would ever show him, but I didn't have the strength to yell at
him to his face, so the next best thing would be to put in writing
the anger that I was feeling.

With each word I wrote I felt guilty for feeling angry but

the anger wouldn't stop. My life, the man I loved, was hanging on to his life in this hospital and I was trying my best to help him. Why and how could this man try and defy the doctors and the nurses who have helped him to stay alive? Why was this man appearing to lose faith in me?

Steve,
I wish I could give you all the things you ask me for. Be it an ice chip, a lollipop, or even a popsicle. Please try to understand that if the doctors are saying no, then they must have a reason.
I have sat at your bedside every day for over a month praying for the Lord to keep you alive and with His help and the help of the doctors they have kept you alive. They saw you through three major surgeries and four minor surgeries. I could have spent the past month next to the bed of a man in a coma, or a man who was totally paralyzed. Worse than that, I could have been kneeling in tears beside a grave.
All these things were risks and possibilities you faced.
But none of them happened.
Now you are on the road to recovery and I have to abide with what they tell me. And if that means saying no to you,
then I am sorry.
I love you too much to do anything that could possibly result in a set back of ANY KIND!!!
Please understand and if you can't then at least know that I am only doing this because I have to and because I love you more than ever.

I closed my notebook and put it away. I would probably not have the heart to let him read it now. I prayed that tomorrow the trachea would come out. Maybe if he could vocalize his feelings then both I and the doctors would be able to give him what he needed.

Still June 23rd.

They took the stitches out on the top of his head. He looks good.

Central line finally out on shoulder.

Dr. Leng said he could have an ice chip if he promised not to swallow it.

PM

Ran fever up to 102 degrees.

Probably means that the trachea won't be changed tomorrow.

WEDNESDAY JUNE 24, 1992

Temperature down to 99 with Motrin.
Walked down to the lounge and sat for a while.
Trachea – hopefully tomorrow.
Dr. Leng in – will try to take missed stitches
out when she has a chance.
Asked her if I should take any precautions with the
shunt at home or when he goes back to work. She
suggested a hard hat.
Went to Spaulding and had a tour. Seems like a nice
place and easy enough to get to. They encourage patients'
spouses to participate in the rehabilitation process. It
would depend on Steve's reaction. Whether or not he
would be distracted with me there or not.
The fever is due to a urinary tract infection.

Steve and I took a walk down to the lounge. I told him all about Spaulding and what they had to offer. I had to let him know that it was not as modern as Mass. General was, however the facilities were nice and I felt that it would do him a lot of good.

Part of him didn't understand why he had to go there but he knew that in order to go home he had to suffer through it. In my heart, I knew that he needed to go.

He tapped me on the shoulder. His lips were trying to form words that I was having a hard time understanding. He slowed down.

"Why didn't you bring my suitcase?" he was trying to ask.

I couldn't believe it. He still thought he had a missing suitcase with white shorts in it. My heart sank. "Honey there is no suitcase. Just like there is no little boy named Utley." My voice was shaking. "You must have dreamt them both."

He slammed his fists down on his knees. "I am not crazy! You all think I am crazy!"

I read those words from his silent lips quite clearly. I made him look me in the eyes. "You are not crazy. You have been through hell and back. Please trust me. They told me that these things that you are so insistent on are probably dreams that you had while you were in I.C.U."

He tried to speak again, "But they seemed so real." The tears were filling up in his eyes. "I can see them as clear as day."

I wish that someone could have given me the words to say to him. There was nothing I could say or do other than to just hold him and let him know that I was there. That I loved him. That soon it would be better. Soon it would be over.

I hoped and prayed for an answer. I wanted us to be home.

THURSDAY JUNE 25, 1992

I was hoping that today would be the day that they would decide to change his trachea. It had been so long since I had heard his voice that I wasn't sure any more what he sounded like.

I called the nurses station to see how he had been during the night. His temperature didn't go above 99.6 all night. When I got to the hospital I stopped to talk to Leanne before going in to see him. She seemed hopeful that it would still be a go for today.

Steve was sitting up in his chair waiting for me. His sneakers were on. He wanted to take a walk down to the lounge. It was so nice to walk with him. I would hold onto one arm while we walked. Even though the nurses were supposed to be with him for the first few days of him being up and around, they were comfortable enough with me now knowing that I was with him to help. I was able to disconnect his feeding tube if he needed to get out of bed. I would be sure to put the salve on his lips and gums to prevent them from getting dried out from lack of use. I started to do the small nursing duties. It did me a lot of good to be able to help him, even if it was just the little things. In a way it helped out the nurses and Steve seemed to appreciate the fact that it was his wife doing some of the private chores.

Temp stayed down all night – right around 99.6
Leanne, (Steve's nurse) feels it will be a go with the
new trachea. Steve is still doing great. We walked
down to the lounge again. Got him some ice chips.
I've really started helping with the little things. Steve
thinks I should get a job as a nurse's aide.
I don't think so. The only reason I do it is to help Steve.

As I was leaving the floor to go downstairs for lunch, I ran into the doctors who would be testing Steve to see if they could change the trachea. They told me to be back in about twenty minutes or so and they would be done.

Twenty minutes!?! Was it really going to happen today? I got on the elevator and went downstairs. I couldn't eat. I was so excited.

I went outside and had a couple of cigarettes. I couldn't wait. I went back upstairs and stood outside his room. The curtain was drawn around his bed. I could hear the doctor giving his assistant instructions.

"Are you okay?" It was Leanne. She was standing beside me looking very concerned.

"Yeah, they might be changing his trachea." My voice was shaky.

"Stay here, I'll see what's going on," she said.

She went in and disappeared around the curtain. A moment later she came back with a smile on her face. "They are doing it right now. It will be another few minutes. If you want to wait in the lounge, I'll come and get you."

"Okay." I didn't want to leave. I wanted to be there when they were done. I wanted to be there when he started to speak. I guess a small part of me was afraid that he might have some speech problem. Worse that he may not be able to speak at all. For the most part though, I was being selfish. I want to be the first one he spoke to. I felt I deserved it.

I walked into the lounge, but I couldn't sit still. I paced for about five minutes before giving up and going back to stand vigil outside his door. When I got back, not only was Leanne standing at the end of his bed, but another nurse, Lisa, was there as well. Lisa saw me and came out.

"They are almost done. You must be so psyched!!" she exclaimed.

All I could do was nod. How was it that they could stand there and his wife had to wait? Why was it that when he first was able to speak, that I was left out here?

Finally I hear the doctor say "Give us a big 'Hello' Steve."

Someone made a sound, I heard the word hello being said by someone. The voice was unfamiliar. Was it Steve?

I started to slowly go in. I looked at Leanne. She smiled with tears in her eyes, and asked the doctor if I could come in.

"I guess there is someone else who wants to hear how you're doing" he said.

I came around the curtain. I could tell the trachea was different and watched as the doctors gathered their instruments.

The doctor turned to Steve and said, "Well, Mr. Merrow, thank you for being such a patient patient." He held out his hand to shake Steve's.

"Thanks Doc." Steve said.

My knees buckled and Leanne grabbed my arm. I reached out for the end of his bed. He was okay. He could talk and he was okay.

"I'm okay Leanne," I whispered.

"Hi princess," Steve said. His voice was soft, but golden to my ears.

"I think they should be alone." Leanne said and took Lisa's arm and they left.

I sat down on Steve's bed, put my head down on his chest and started to cry. He held on to me and when I looked up at his face, he was crying too.

"It's about time," was all he said, then he lifted my head and looked at me. "I love you princess" and he held me tight.

They changed his trachea. Thank you God!
It was so good to hear him talk.

I cried, he cried, the nurses cried.
When I got back from shopping for Dawn's birthday
present tonight, there was a message on my mothers
answering machine. It was from Steve!
Called him at the hospital twice. Almost to make
sure that he could still say I love you.

That night I went shopping for Dawn's birthday present. I would be going home this weekend to celebrate her fifth birthday. I needed to have something special. I spotted it in the toy aisle. A child's tape recorder! It was perfect. Tomorrow I would bring it with me to the hospital and let Steve record a message for Dawn. I picked up a couple of story book tapes to go along with it and a blank cassette.

When I got home that night I saw that there was a message on my mother's answering machine. I rewound the tape and pressed play. "Hi...it's me...call me back when you get home....bye!"

My Mom and Dad looked at me funny. I played it back again. Then it hit me who it was on the phone. Steve! My heart was jumping for joy. I grabbed the phone and called his room. It was so good to be able to talk to him. It made me realize that he was definitely on his way back to me.

FRIDAY JUNE 26, 1992

I had one day left with Steve before I would go home to the kids for the weekend. I wanted to spend as much time with him as I could. It was heaven to be able to talk to him without trying to either read his lips or to decipher his handwriting. We took walks up and down the corridor and down to the lounge. He finally convinced a nurse to let me take him outside to the courtyard.

He knew that his next hurdle was to build up his strength enough for them to transfer him to Spaulding and then home.

Steve was getting stronger, too. He used the walker, but only to appease the nurses. He carried it more than he used it for support. The wheelchair was only used to get him from his room to the courtyard. His legs did most of the work.

His physical appearance was fine. The scars on his face were minor and in time would probably be very hard to see.

We found a scale during one of our walks and Steve stepped on. It showed that since all of this started he lost forty five pounds. He was now down to one hundred and eighty five pounds. The weight didn't bother me. I knew that once they allowed him to eat he would put it back on in no time.

His left eye was still a problem. It would not turn to the left any more than a fraction of an inch. I had picked him up an eye patch at the local pharmacy and that helped him out but without it covered he constantly saw double.

His only request to me for when I went home was to bring in my barber shears and finish the haircut the surgeons had started. He only had a half a head of hair and wanted me to even it out for him.

We talked a lot about what has happened to him and the different procedures they had done to him. The conversations were very emotional to say the least. He insisted on being told as much as I could tell him. He didn't want me to leave him alone for the weekend but he knew that I had to be with Dawn for her birthday. He tried to put a message on her tape recorder for her but couldn't get more than a "happy birthday" and an "I love you" out.

Temperature still down.
Bacteria found in the culture taken from a lumbar
puncture...probably a contaminant from the skin.
They put him on antibiotics anyway to be safe.

Four walks down to the lounge and two trips out to
the courtyard.

Still no word on when he can have real food.
Snuck lollipops from my purse.
Temperature at ninety eight point nine tonight.

SATURDAY JUNE 27, 1992

Temperature at 98.5 degrees.
Cat scan today or tomorrow
Dawn's birthday today. Called Steve and got the kids
on the phone.
Dawn wanted to cry when she heard Daddy's
voice and Happy Birthday message on her new tape
recorder.

Called the hospital off and on during the day to talk to
Steve.
Marybeth came by the house. Stayed all day.
Tammy 'Mighty Moe' came by for Dawn's party. She had
a card with all kinds of checks from the women I had
worked with at the bank.
Sometimes I feel like I am so alone and then I realize how
many people I have around me. Not only trying to hold me
up and help me through this, but making sure that Steve
will be okay by doing things and giving things in order to
financially help out and ease his worries.

People helping people.

SATURDAY P.M.
Talked to Steve at about nine-thirty or so.
I thought coming home would be easier this time
because I would be able to talk to him during the
day, but all it did was make me realize even more
that he's not here.
Peg and Bill went in to see him. They talked to him in
detail about the day of the surgery.
No cat scan today.

SUNDAY JUNE 28, 1992

My parents had come home with me this time. I could tell when they woke up that they were tired and worn out. They were not used to the routine and madness that a house with four children can bring.

Danielle and Jimmy were going to their fathers house for a few days. Dawn and Becky were going to go to Linda Grant's house.

I cleaned the house and got everybody packed. After the two older kids were on their way, I took the two younger ones over to Linda's. From there, my parents brought me back to the hospital.

When I walked into his room he was sitting up in his bed. His feet were donned with socks and sneakers. He wanted to go outside to the courtyard. I had no sooner put my things down and helped him to his feet when in walked his younger sister, Diane, with her fiancée, Keith. They went outside with us and we all sat in the sun. It was a very nice visit. We sat out there for about an hour. They said their goodbyes and I took Steve back upstairs. Once in his room Steve asked if I remembered the barber shears. My mind went back to that morning when I was tearing the house apart looking for them.

Steve had called in the midst of the chaos and when I told him that I was having trouble finding them, he knew right were they were. It was hard to believe that he was the one in the hospital after undergoing brain surgery, and I had to have him remember where things were in the house.

It only took about twenty minutes to "style" his hair. It was not perfect because I was nervous cutting near the scars and the shunt. Once it was done though he not only looked better, but he felt better too.

I sat down next to him on the bed. He smiled back at me. I asked him if I could get a hug from him, but before he could answer me his mother and her friend Tom were coming into the room.

I got up off of the bed and let his mother come over to say hello. They visited for about an hour. During that time, I went downstairs and got Steve a newspaper and a soda for everyone. Steve walked to the lounge for a little while before his mother left.

As his mother was saying her goodbyes to Steve, and Steve was doing his best to reassure her that he would be okay, Marybeth came in to visit.

I looked at Steve and smiled. Marybeth sat down for a few minutes before Steve decided that he wanted to go back outside to the courtyard.

We sat for about five minutes when Steve wanted to go and sit on the grass. Well, the spot he picked out was on a small incline and he no sooner got out of the wheelchair than his foot slipped out from under him and he landed smack dab on his butt.

He sat there for a moment shaking his head and then he started to laugh. He was fine, but my heart was in my throat. I wanted to hit him for laughing but at least he was all right.

Marybeth went inside to get an apple juice for me and herself. When she came back, Steve put his hand out.

"What do you think you're doing?" I asked him.

"Come on, honey, I only want a sip. It won't hurt me. I drink the melted ice water. Just one sip. That's all I want. Just one. Please?"

How could I refuse him? His one sip turned into about half the can.

Marybeth and I took him back upstairs before she had to go. I looked at Steve and told him that I was going to walk her outside.

"Sure...you only want to go and have a cigarette." He smiled.

"I will be right back."

It was more than that though. Next weekend was the Fourth of July and I needed to know if she could sit with the kids for the weekend.

She didn't even bat an eye. "No problem," she said. No problem for her, but I was getting a massive case of the guilts. So many people had done so much for me. She told me to be quiet. She was turning out to be such a good friend. One of the best friends I had.

Marybeth, Linda and Sue had all taken so much of their time to help me get through all of this. As I tried to explain this to Marybeth, as I tried to let her know that they all meant so much to me I could feel myself wanting to cry again.

Marybeth, straight shooter that she is, said, "Knock off the shit. That's what friends are for."

She gave me a big hug and took off.

I finished my cigarette and went back up to Steve. He was waiting for me and the two of us went out to the lounge to sit. I helped him manage his IV pole around the sofa and then sat down next to him.

"Alone at last," he said and put his arm around my shoulder.

I snuggled up against him and lifted my face to his. In the corner of my mind, I could hear the bell of the elevator. Steve bent his head to kiss me.

"Break it up you two," a voice bellowed from behind us. "You're in a hospital you know."

It was my Dad. He wanted to come in early to get me so that he could spend some time with Steve.

I couldn't believe it. After about twenty minutes, Dad went downstairs to wait for me to allow Steve and I some 'quiet' time together.

I looked at Steve and laughed. He gave me a big hug and kissed me.

"I love you," he told me.

"I love you too." More than he'll ever know

No ct-scan today.
BP still good.
Temperature at 98.5

MONDAY JUNE 29, 1992

We were told that they had to do a ct-scan before Steve would be able to go to Spaulding. I couldn't understand why it had not been done yet. Steve was getting so frustrated. He knew that he had to regain a lot of strength back. He knew that at Spaulding they would be able to help him do that. I knew at Spaulding they would be able to prepare him for what was ahead of him.

> *Dr. Joseph in to see Steve this morning*
> *Remember: bone missing in area behind nasal passages*
> *No doctors are to go through his nose other than Dr. Joseph*
> *or Dr. Ogilvy.*
> *Ear tubes are temporary and will come out on their own.*
> *CT-scan better be done today.*

Steve had me call Dr. Ogilvy's office in the afternoon. He wanted to know when he would be scheduled for the ct-scan. The doctor was in surgery, but the secretary told me that she would let him know Steve's concern and that she would call me back as soon as she could.

By the time I was ready to go home we found out that he was now scheduled for the scan that night. Steve and I just smiled at each other. We knew why. Dr. Ogilvy had come through for us again.

> *Temperature at 98.7*
> *Steve is doing really well. I haven't seen any confusion in*
> *days.*

Not on the blood pressure medication any longer? I will ask about

that. He was given strong antibiotic for the last time. Temperature

stayed down all day. Linda Grant may visit.

Called the doctor's office to talk to Dr. Ogilvy. He was in OR. Told the secretary that we wanted to know why the CT scan had not been

done yet. She said she would have the doctor look into it and get

back to us.

CT scan now on for tonight! Steve back by 7:45. Linda and Robert Grant and myself went to see him. It was a good visit. Dr. O. in to see Steve at ten o'clock. Said CT showed the clips were exposed. What does that mean?

TUESDAY JUNE 30, 1992

We talked a lot about Steve going to Spaulding. We were told that it would happen within the next week. Steve was very anxious. He wanted to be there and then on his way home. We waited for the day that he got the okay to eat food. It drove him crazy that people in the bed next to him could eat and he couldn't.

> *Steve called at quarter to eight this morning and said that*
> *Dr. Joseph was in. The Dr. said that the fact that the clips*
> *were exposed could be a problem. Could delay his eating.*
> *What does that mean??*
> *Will it delay him from going to Spaulding?(ANSWER: No.*
> *If they have to they will send him with the feeding tube.)*
> *Will the clips cover over by themselves? (ANSWER: Yes.)*

I wasn't going to the hospital until later in the morning. Steve called me back at about eight o'clock to tell me that he had an appointment at Dr. Joseph's office at nine o'clock and that from there he was going over to have someone look at his eye.

I told Steve to find out how the clips were exposed. I told him to find out what-that meant. He told me to calm down. That he would see me when I got to the hospital.

I went around the house and cleaned up for my Mom. Before I left for the hospital I tried to call Dr. Joseph myself to find out about the clips. The nurse put me on hold and when the phone was answered, it wasn't the nurse, and it wasn't the doctor. It was Steve.

"Hi!" he said, very matter of factly. "Trachea is gone."

"What?" I didn't understand how that could be.

"Dr. Joe took out the trachea. My swallow test was easy. He gave me a cup of coffee, I drank it, and he said okay. That was it."

I looked up at the clock. The next bus would be here in ten minutes. "I am on my way in."

I flew on a cloud all the way there. When I arrived at the hospital, he was still not back yet but they expected him at any moment.

I went to the lounge to wait.

Steve is still at Mass. Eye and Ear having his eye looked at. I've been here a while waiting, very impatiently. Bumped into Dr. Leng on the elevator. She said the plan is for him to go to Spaulding tomorrow.
So our stay here at Mass. General is coming to a close.
It is so remarkable how far Steve has come. When I think of him not being able to open his eyes or talk and then the fight came. He stunned everyone. He showed them all he was not one to stay down.

Later in the afternoon, a social worker came in to let us know that Steve would be going to the rehab tomorrow.

As soon as she left the room, Steve and I held on to each other and cried. It was finally going to happen. What was once only a dream, was now about to come true.

That night, I went home and called everyone. Steve is going to Spaulding tomorrow!

It is finally official...Spaulding here he comes.
Warm up the weights and heat up the food.
Steve is getting ready to come home.

The trachea is out.
Someone at Mass. Eye and Ear looked at his eyes...dilated them.

The optic nerve was nicked during surgery. Worst case scenario
is that he wears an eye patch.
Probably have to wear glasses.
Make sure Doctors take out final stitches.

P.M.
I'm on the phone with you. I can't believe that tomorrow is finally here!

It is about midnight. I can't call you. I wish I could. I can't sleep.
I close my eyes and I see everything we have been through. I see
the pain in your eyes. I see the monitors. I feel the heartache all
over again.
It doesn't seem like it's been almost seven weeks since
this nightmare began. I wish you could understand how this
has been for me. I know too much maybe. A nurse once said
it was both good and bad that I understood so much.
Good because when you wanted to know I would be there to
answer your questions. Bad, because I knew exactly what was happening.

I'll tell you though...I have met and talked to people who don't understand, and I think I would rather know.

The hardest part of all will be telling you about the seizures.
You are going to have to accept the fact that it is a possibility
for your future and that you will have to continue on your medication to prevent them.

I am so scared sometimes of waking up and something is going to go wrong. Then I hear the determination you have and I know that everything will be okay.

WEDNESDAY JULY 1, 1992

The ambulance to transport Steve to Spaulding would be at the hospital by nine-thirty so I had to hurry and get ready. They were letting me go over with him on the ambulance and I was not about to be late. I also was not going to get on a bus with an empty suitcase. The taxi was outside beeping at eight-thirty. I was there by ten minutes to nine.

When I got to his room he was in the shower. I opened the suitcase and started to pack his belongings. I took all the cards down off the wall. There must have been about fifty or more. I packaged them up and put them in a manila envelope. I gathered all of the clothes that he had been accumulating. All of the stuffed animals, except for George, went into the suitcase. George would be riding with us.

I heard the shower turn off. A few moments later Steve opened the bathroom door and stepped out. When I looked at him, I got an uneasy feeling. He looked very pale. As he got closer, I noticed that he was shaking as well.

"I'm really cold, have you packed my bathrobe yet?" he asked.

I took it out and wrapped it around his shoulders. "Do you feel okay?" I put my hand up towards his forehead in an attempt to see if he had a fever, but he pulled away.

"I'm fine honey," he said. "I just took a shower and I'm chilly, that's all."

He was making me nervous. He got dressed and we took a walk down to the lounge to wait.

"Can you rub the back of my neck? I must have slept funny or something last night."

"Are you sure you're okay?" I asked. He did not look good at all.

"No, I don't think I feel very good. Don't tell anybody. There is not going to be anything to get in the way of me leaving this place today."

"Okay. I won't tell them, but I think you should tell them yourself. It won't mean that you won't go. They have doctors over there too. They can treat you over there just as well as they can treat you here." He was starting to feel a little warm to me. I was afraid that he was starting to run a fever.

"I don't care," he was saying, "Just don't say anything to them."

I gave him my word.

We went back to his room. He wanted to lie down for a little bit before they showed up. The nurse was walking down to get us anyway.

"Mr. Merrow, I need to examine you for the last time so that I can sign you out." She walked the rest of the way back to his room with us.

He lay down on the bed and the nurse started to do her thing. First she checked his blood pressure. It was a little bit elevated, but she said he was probably anxious about the transfer. She checked his pulse and then she stuck a thermometer in his mouth. He was running a low grade temperature. He had the chills as well.

She threw another blanket over him and stepped out of the room. While she was out, I noticed that the paramedics were outside of Steve's room. The nurse whispered something to one of them and came back into the room.

"Steve, I've put a call into Dr. Yu to come up to look at you. You are running a low grade temperature and I would feel better if he examined you before I sign you out." She felt his forehead again before leaving. She turned back to us before she left the room. "This doesn't mean anything. I just want to be sure."

"I don't believe this," Steve said. "I just want to go home and see my kids." He was shivering. The look in his eyes was simply heartbreaking.

"I'm so sorry Steve." I sat down on his bed and put my arms around him.

A few minutes later I went out to the nurses' station. The paramedics were waiting patiently. One of them looked at me and asked me how long we had been here.

I told her that it seemed like forever, but that we had been there for almost two months. She put her hand on my shoulder and said that things would be fine.

I saw Dr. Yu come down the hall. He stopped quickly to talk to Steve's nurse and went in to examine him. He wasn't in there for more than two or three minutes. I heard him tell Steve, "Just a couple of days. We'll get you out of here. Don't worry."

> *I feel so bad. You worked so hard for this. Please don't hurt*
> *too bad. One or two days.*
> *Temperature at 99.8*
> *Blood Pressure 150 over 90*
> *Pulse rate 112*
> *Chills*
> *No discharge from here for him today.*
>
> *Not realized until EMT's were at the door to get him.*
>
> *I am so sorry. I know the only reason you said anything*
> *To the doctor was because I was worried.*
> *I know how much this must be hurting you because*
> *My heart is breaking in two. I am so sorry.*

Steve kept complaining about his neck hurting. By two o'clock that afternoon his temperature was up to 102. The doctor ordered a lumbar puncture. He thought it might be spinal meningitis. The chills only got worse. Steve was so very sick and I felt so very helpless.

> *2:00... Temp up to 102*
> *Lumbar puncture to be done – could be spinal meningitis*

What is happening?
God...please help him.

His fever just kept going up. The nurses started to take his temp every twenty minutes or so.

2:15 – temp at 103.1
2:45 – temp at 104

All hell broke loose. If they didn't get the fever down and get it down fast, Steve could start having seizures. They gave him a shot of Phenobarbital to keep that from happening.

I was terrified to leave the room. I felt so helpless, again. I looked down at Steve. He was still shivering. "I am so sorry." I said to him. My eyes were filling up with tears.

"I am so sick this time," Steve said. "I can't believe this is happening. It's just not fair."

"I know, but at least it happened here. If you got to Spaulding and this happened, they would have had to send you back." I knew it was little consolation, but it was true.

Just then a nurse came into the room with a basin of ice and a bottle of alcohol.

"We have to get your fever to go down, Steve," she said. "This is going to be miserable but please bear with us."

She poured the alcohol into the basin along with his pitcher of water. She then went back out of the room and came back with a handful of towels. She handed me half of them and told me to do what she did. One by one we soaked the towels into the icy solution and then placed them on his legs, his arms, his chest and his stomach. One was even wrapped around his head like a turban. Two other nurses kept coming in with more buckets filled with ice to help. We filled ice packs and placed them under his armpits and under his knees.

He was so good about the whole thing. He just lay there while the nurses and I rotated the towels and kept his body iced.

Within an hour or so we had his temperature forced down to 101.9.

The ice bath stopped but the nurse warned me that the fever would rise back on its own. They needed to locate the source of the infection and treat it. They started to pump him with antibiotics.

A doctor came in and performed a lumbar puncture on him. She told me I could stay. Maybe with me there, he would not stir and they would only have to do it once. It was such a miserable test to do. The fever had knocked so much out of Steve. He slept through the entire procedure.

I called my father and asked him to pick me up at about six o'clock. When I left, his temperature had gone down to about 100.6.

Checked with the P.M. nurse at about 8:00 – temp at about 100.4
She told me that a cisternogram was planned for tomorrow. Why!!

I have to call Dr. Ogilvy.

I was panic stricken. A cisternogram was such an ordeal that if it had been ordered for tomorrow then the doctor was looking for a leak. I knew that much. I asked the nurse on the phone if she had told Steve. She had only told him the fact that there was a test scheduled in radiology but hadn't told him everything. I told her that when he was awake to have him call me. I wanted to be the one tell him.

She didn't know anything about why though. She suggested that I call his doctor if I was that concerned.

Dr. Ogilvy says that the count in the spinal fluid is high.
Which means the infection is probably spinal meningitis.
He also says that there could be a leak that could be causing the spinal meningitis.
The cisternogram would let them know if the leak is there,

how bad it is, and if it will mean more surgery. He said that
he wanted me to be prepared IN CASE he needed to be
operated
on again in order to repair it.

For this doctor to say these things to me made me feel as
though he was certain that there was a leak. After all that we
have had to go through, why else would he scare me this way.

Dear God, how much more can he endure? How much
more will he have to take? How much more CAN he take?

THURSDAY JULY 2, 1992

I called his morning nurse, Karen, and arranged with her to be allowed into his room early in the morning. I called a taxi and got to the hospital by nine o'clock that morning. This test, the cisternogram, was miserable, and I wanted to be with Steve when he had to go down. He had been through it before but doesn't remember any of it. He was very scared and needed me to be with him.

I wouldn't be allowed into radiology with him but was able to go with him as far as the entrance. They in turn left him on the transport bed to wait.

"This is jus so unfair," he said to me. There were tears in his eyes. No one could blame him for being upset. This had hit him hard and so fast. He wanted so badly to be at Spaulding. He only wanted to go home.

I had no answers for him. I just held his hand. His other hand was gripping his stuffed animal, George.

A doctor came over to us and wheeled Steve into a room down the corridor. He pulled me aside and went over the procedure and told me all the risks involved.

"You've been through this before, you know that I need you to sign a consent form. It's just routine." He reached out his hand and tried to hand me a pen.

I looked at the form and then up at the doctor. "My husband is the one who should have to sign this. He is quite capable of using a pen and I think you should be telling him the risks of this whole thing. It is his body, and his life that you are dealing with, not mine." I couldn't believe that I had said that.

I knew though, that I was right. I reached up and handed him back the consent form.

I was asked to come in with the doctor so that I would know the rest of the procedure. When I walked through the door I saw that they had put Steve into "position". He had been put onto a table at a forty five degree angle. His feet were bound with leather straps that held him and kept him from slipping. His head was at the lower end of the table.

They explained how an injection of contrast dye would be injected into his spine and would travel to his brain. They would then take him into the CT-scan room and take pictures of his brain. The entire time however, he would have to remain at a slight angle without lifting his head for about an hour.

I hadn't told Steve my fears about surgery. I never told him that Dr. Ogilvy was looking for a leak. He thought this test had to do with the meningitis. I didn't want to scare him any more than he already was. I had no idea of how I would tell him anyway.

Temp not below 101 during the night.
AM nurse – Karen
In the morning it was at 99.8
IV started last night
On a cooling blanket
Complaining of a headache and a stiff neck
Not showing any signs of confusion

I stayed with him all day. The test took a little bit over an hour to complete. He was so tired. This was because of the fever they told me. He slept most of the morning and into the afternoon.

I was very anxious to hear the results of the test. I kept after the nurse all day. Finally she took out his chart and read what the radiologist had noted.

"CSF flowed freely by the basilar artery," she read.

"That's fine," I said. "What I need to know though is

what the fluid does after it passes the basilar artery. Does it say anything else? Does it say anything about a leak?"

There was nothing written. She told me that as soon as one of Steve's doctors came onto the floor she would have them call down to radiology.

That seemed to take forever. At about four o'clock, I spotted a doctor referred to as "Dr. Jane" at the nurses station. I went out to her and asked her if she would call radiology for me.

As she made her call, I paced between the nurses station and Steve's bed. Steve was sleeping. Finally she put the receiver down and approached me. We were right outside Steve's room.

My hands were shaking and I had a lump in my throat. I had been trying all day to prepare myself for this moment. It didn't seem to matter. The doctor looked at me and asked if I was okay.

"What did they say," I asked her.

She looked at me and smiled, "No leak!"

I started to cry and a voice came out of Steve's room. "Hey you guys! I thought I was the patient here. Does somebody want to come in here and tell me what the hell is going on?"

I went in to him and told him, "There was no leak on the CT-scan they did. You are okay."

"I know that," he said, "Why are you crying?"

"Because I was afraid that you might have surgery again. The doctor had told me last night that if they found a leak, they would have to open you back up and operate." I told him what the doctor had said and what I had been going through all day.

He was angry at me that I hadn't told him. But the relief I suppose was greater than his anger. He just pulled me to him and held me.

CT-scan showed no leak!!!
So no surgery....
Temp still down.
He has spinal meningitis.

The next couple of days were spent pumping Steve with his antibiotics and getting him back on his feet. I didn't want him to stay in bed for fear that he would lose the strength in his legs again. He had worked so hard to lose anything else at this point.

He still complained of headaches but the doctors all said that it was due to the meningitis. Dr. Joseph followed up with a bedside exam and told us that everything looked good.

His stomach tube, the G-tube came out and he was given the okay to eat solid food. My Dad surprised him with an order of fried scallops. It was terrific to watch him enjoy real food. I doubt that scallops were ever enjoyed more.

The heartache was there but the determination to get himself back on his feet and on his way to Spaulding was greater. He told me that he would be home by July fifteenth. I wanted so much to believe him but that decision would be made from the doctors at Spaulding.

I didn't say anything to Steve. I couldn't bear to see him disappointed anymore. I only prayed each night that God would give him the answers he wanted. That a doctor would sign his release soon to go to Spaulding.

FRIDAY JULY 3, 1992

Dr. Joseph in – looks good.
Temp at 98.8
Headache.
I have to get him up and out of bed.
He has to keep using his legs.

I am so tired.....

Steve just called...He was so psyched!
He had a hard poo!!!

Steve slept a lot. Dad brought him
Scallops. G – Tube came out.

SATURDAY JULY 4, 1992

Spoke to Steve a little while ago.
I wish this was his Independence Day!

Everything still going well.

Waited for the fireworks (from the esplanade)
They finally cancelled them.

Went home by eleven PM

Hurt my back in the shower.

SUNDAY JULY 5, 1992

*Didn't get any sleep last night. My back
was killing me. I can't go in to the hospital today.*

*Called Steve. Told him my back was sore from falling
and I wouldn't be able to see him today.*

*He keeps calling looking for me. I feel so guilty for not going
in. He is okay though. He will be fine.*

I'm going in.

*Saw the fireworks with him from his room. Took a couple
of
nice walks.*

*I miss him so much. I need him to hold me and kiss me
because I am starting to feel so alone.*

I need him so badly.

MONDAY JULY 6, 1992

All vital signs still good.
Will stay on IV instead of being switched to
antibiotics in pill form
Very angry and frustrated about IV and
everything else in general.

His temper was getting the best of him and making just about everyone else miserable. He was mad about the fact that they wouldn't take him off the IV. He was mad because no one was talking to him about going to Spaulding. He was in such a miserable mood that it seemed that everything and everybody was going to set him off. I didn't know what to do.

I offered to call his social worker, Judy, and see if she might have an idea of when he would be transferred but she was not in today. When I told Steve that, however, he insisted that I call Dr. Ogilvy's office and see if he could stop in today to see him. All the secretary could do was take the message and do her best. Not having the doctor be available only made things worse.

Looking for Judy S. – Social Worker
She has the day off.
Called Social Services. They will make sure
That Judy stops in to Steve in the morning.
Called Dr. Ogilvy's office. Steve wants to see him.

I was at my wits end. I didn't know what to do to calm him down. It was about three o'clock when I was passing the nurses station. Someone was on the phone and I heard them mention Steve's name. I asked one of the nurses who the woman was on the phone. I was told that she was a social worker. They must have sent her up to review Steve's file.

I went back into his room but I didn't dare say anything to him about the social worker. I couldn't get his hopes up. I started to pace.

It seemed like an eternity, but about ten minutes later she came into the room.

"Mr. Merrow? How are you feeling today?" She introduced herself and explained that she had been reviewing his medical chart. "It seems that you are doing much better than you were a week ago!"

"You can say that again," he replied. "Can I go to Spaulding?"

"Well as a matter of fact, providing your fever stays away, I have arranged for you to be transferred there tomorrow. Is that soon enough?"

Yes! I wanted to shout it from the rooftops! But not my husband. Always trying to get the last word in on things, he gave out a heavy sigh and said, "Well, I'd rather it be today, but I guess I don't have much of a choice."

She went over a few things with us and then shook Steve's hand before leaving.

"Good luck, Mr. Merrow."

I looked at Steve. "I don't believe it. It's almost over."

"It's about time," he said and put his arms around me.

He didn't want me calling everyone this time. He wanted to be sure he was there first.

Social worker on the floor about three o'clock.
I heard her on the phone with someone and she was
talking about Steve.
When she got off the phone she said that he was
going to Spaulding tomorrow!
As long as there is no fever.

TUESDAY JULY 7, 1992

I didn't sleep a wink. I thought about everything. I was so scared that Steve's fever would come back. That something would happen to keep him from going. Steve told me not to worry, that everything would be fine. That he felt great and that nothing, but nothing would get in his way this time.

Steve called the house at seven o'clock. He said he felt great. No chills, no headache, no neck aches, and that his stomach was fine.

Steve's only concern was the fact that he had a bad problem controlling his bladder at night. The nurses and the doctors told us that it was due to the fact that all the medications that he was on wiped him out and he simply slept too soundly. It was something that in time would simply stop. Yet being the type of man Steve is, this was a major problem and was worse than the fear of any future seizures. When we got home, I had the feeling that it would stop. If not, then before that.

I got to the hospital early in order to accompany him on the ambulance. I made sure that everything was packed.

Aside from being a little nervous, Steve was fine. He was so excited about leaving. It was almost unreal to think that his hospital stay had come to an end. To think that within a few weeks, he would be home.

The paramedics weren't there until eleven o'clock. They had to strap him onto a transport bed. He hated that so much. He even went so far as to ask if he could walk over. He tried to have them take him in a wheel chair van. His reasoning was that he didn't want to leave the same way he came in. They compromised and raised the head of the bed so that he was sitting up.

They wheeled him out into the hall. Every nurse on the floor came over to see him and to wish him luck. There were a few with tears in their eyes. It was so touching to watch. Karen and Tamsan came to me and gave me a big hug.

Even Dr. Gress came over from I.C.U. and shook Steve's hand. Then he turned to me and gave me a hug. "I told you once before and I meant it. The hard part is just about to start for you. Make sure you keep up on your rest and remember that you are not only taking care of him, but yourself too."

I thanked him for all of his help and his support. He was a good doctor and had become a good friend to both of us.

We were on our way. The ambulance ride took about five minutes. When they "unloaded" him they stopped at the admitting office. We signed him in and then we went up to the sixth floor and Steve's new room.

The décor left something to be desired but it didn't matter. To both of us this was nothing more than a stop over until he went home.

The nurse that came in to take his vitals was amazed at the condition he was in. She told us that she expected a patient that was going to need help getting out of bed. That when she had read his file and saw the type of surgery he had undergone that she thought he would be a lot worse.

No sooner had we started to get Steve unpacked than a woman by the name of Lynn entered the room. She introduced herself as Steve's physical therapist.

She started to explain the routine he would be going through when an Asian woman dressed in a white jacket came in. She shook Steve's hand and told us her name was Dr. Woo. She would be observing his first session with Lynn in order to start her evaluation of him.

We all went down to the physical therapy room. While Lynn started with Steve, Dr. Woo sat with me.

"How is it going?" she asked me.

"He's doing fine," I replied.

"That's not what I meant, I was asking how you are doing. This whole thing must be taking its toll on you as well as on Steve." She seemed so concerned. She was such a nice woman.

I told her how I had been coping and about how I have been staying with my parents. That I missed my kids. That they wanted us both to be back at home.

"When do you think you would want him home," she asked me.

"Well, I wanted him home yesterday. I wish I could take him home now. But I know that he needs to be stronger. I need for him to be okay."

The entire time that the two of us were talking she would watch Steve with Lynn. They were going through some simple exercises and balancing maneuvers.

I explained to the doctor that Steve was bothered by his bladder control, or lack of it at night. She asked me what type of medication he had been on. I told her that he took six hundred milligrams of phenobarbitol over the course of the day. She told me that this particular medication would wipe him out and that she was going to change it to tegritol.

When Lynn and Steve were finished Dr. Woo called Steve over. I couldn't believe what happened next.

"Steve, I think you are doing just great. Aside from some need for physical therapy I think you are almost ready to go home." She looked at me and smiled. "Mrs. Merrow, do you think you could handle him being home some time next week?"

I couldn't believe my ears. "Are you sure?"

Steve looked at me. "I'm sure. What day?"

Dr. Woo smiled, "Well, tomorrow is Wednesday, why not shoot for next Wednesday. How does that sound."

"Dynamite," Steve said. "Thank you so much."

Later on that afternoon it hit us. Next Wednesday would be July 15th. The day Steve set as his goal to be home.

TUESDAY JULY 7, 1992 P.M.

So you are at Spaulding!!
They brought you by ambulance (much to your dismay)
at about eleven thirty this morning.
All the nurses, Karen, Tamsen, Irini and even Dr. Gress
came to say goodbye and to wish you luck. I was so
emotional.

At Spaulding though was the best. We got you signed in and
the nurses couldn't believe the shape their patient was in.
They expected a very ill patient. You sure impressed them
all!

I can't believe it's almost over.

I called Karen at Mass. General and told her. She was so
psyched!

Your sister Linda had her baby!

Colleen Michelle DeCola. 8 pounds.

What a day. I wish you would finish your cigarette and get
back to your room. I am dying to tell you about your new
God-daughter.

Steve,
We had such a nice talk on the phone last night. I meant
what I said. These past two months have been so hard on
us. Physically and emotionally you have been through hell.

There were times when I thought I would lose you and times when I thought your recovery would not go as well as it has.

Through it all, I had a lot of times when I did nothing but think of us. When I did nothing but remembering everything.

But most of all realizing that I could not live without you. You are my reason for being, my life and my best friend. I never realized how much one person could love another and that love I have for you. I love you more today than yesterday, but not as much as tomorrow.

WEDNESDAY JULY 8, 1992

Had a busy day...and night.

10:00 A.M. – When I got there you were already with your occupational therapists, Karen and Monica. It was a good session. Tested you senses, as far as being able to distinguish from a sharp pin and a dull paper clip. Tested your perception to movement.

11:00 A.M. – On to speech therapy, with Pam, another good session. Asked questions as to why you thought you were here and then testing your memory as far as grammar and usage of the language.

12:00 – Lunch! We dined on Dad's spaghetti.

1:30 P.M. Your support group meeting.

2:00 P.M. – Physical Therapy with Lynn. Simple stretching exercises and then balancing and coordination exercises followed by walking a few flights of stairs and then...the bike.
More stretching and then we went out on the terrace.

Diane came to visit for a while and may come back tomorrow. When I tried to call you the nurse told me your neuro-psych exam was moved from tomorrow to tonight.

You called me to tell me you were back and that you were going to grab a quick smoke and call me back.

I can't wait to hear how it went. I feel that this is an important part of your recovery.

It sounds like it went well. I am so amazed that you are doing so well. Nothing would make me happier than to be in your arms right now.

THURSDAY, JULY 9, 1992

Busy day again.

I spoke with the occupational therapist and with Dr. Woo. The only problem they are seeing is with short term memory and with you putting stupid wooden puzzles together.

I don't see the second as being a problem. I don't think they should either.
The memory could be nothing more than the pressure of being tested.

I am not worried about that either.

I was present for some of the tests that the occupational and speech therapists were giving Steve. Most of them he passed with flying colors. Those were the ones that made sense and applied to everyday life. Some of the tests that I witnessed however I couldn't understand, let alone a man who had undergone what he had. Not only that, but had the added pressure of having to prove to a medical community that he was fit enough to return home.

So I was not concerned when they approached me and told me that further therapy in these areas would be needed after he was released.

I spoke to Dr. Woo. She seemed to understand where I was coming from. After all, I was his wife, I knew him better than they did and I wasn't worried about it.

She also told me the things to watch for, such as sudden mood swings. She also told me that they would all sit down and review his entire case before releasing him.

FRIDAY JULY 10, 1992

Physical therapy – 2 sessions
Went good.
Occupational Therapy – went well.

Speech Therapy –
Spoke with Pam for a minute while Steve was taking a
test.
I never realized that the area where the aneurysm was
located
was in the part of the brain that controls the memory. The
fact that there is a problem with short term memory is
very understandable. I guess he is lucky that the long term
memory
was not affected.

I talked with his Speech Therapist for about five minutes while she was having Steve take a test.

"Not for nothing Pam, but he has told me about some of the tests that you and others have had him do. He feels that he has to prove himself to all of you and it is probably making him very nervous. I don't think I could pass some of the tests that you give him, even under easier conditions."

"Lauri, you yourself have told me occasions that he has forgotten things. He didn't remember my name after a couple of hours. We need to know how badly his short term memory has been affected."

That was when I found out that the aneurysm was located

near the portion of the brain that controls your memory. Pam showed me a diagram and pointed out where the leak was and how the blood and fluid that collected in that area deadened some of the tissue of the brain.

I stopped her, "Pam, it was Steve a few weeks ago that had to tell me over the phone where something was located at home after I had spent hours looking for it." I was recalling the barber shears, and how I couldn't find them that morning.

"I don't think his long term memory is a problem. He does not do well at any of the tests involving his short term memory. What happens if a customer tells him what they want and he forgets when he is halfway down the aisle to get it? Or if he forgets the price of a piece of lumber? We need to work with him on ways to help himself in those areas."

I understood what she was saying but felt in my heart that once Steve was home that those things would work themselves out. He felt pressured here. He felt he had something to prove here. As well he did.

FRIDAY JULY 10, 1992 – after therapy

Now that Steve is at Spaulding, things are moving along so much faster. It is as though now he is facing the final stretch and is going to sprint to the finish line. He can't seem to get enough. He finishes one therapy session and wants to move right on to the next one. He is the most determined man I have ever seen. His determination will only get him home to us that much faster.

All of his therapists encourage me to participate in his sessions. Lynn, his physical therapist, has me doing the exercises right along with him. Right down to riding the exercise bike a couple of miles a day. Now at least I feel as though I am actually participating in this unrelenting effort to help him recover.

Each day sees him getting stronger, not only physically, but emotionally as well. He is amazing everyone.

Dr. Woo told us that Steve would be allowed to take the day off on Saturday. That he would be able to leave the hospital and spend the day with me. I was so excited about being able to have a day with him away from all the doctors, and the nurses and the hectic routine that Steve underwent every day.

When the doctor told us about it the first thing I did was ask her what he could do and if there would be any restrictions put on him.

She looked at me and smiled, "He will be able to do anything he wants to."

I laughed, "Where is the closest Holiday Inn?"

I was only joking, but I guess they took me quite seriously, "There is one right near Mass. General, but keep in mind that you only have the day, he has to be back here at the end of the day."

I looked at Steve, who was smiling, I never thought about being able to make love to him before he had been released from here. The idea scared me. I knew that he would want to, but I wasn't sure if it was safe or not. In the mean time the doctor and the therapists were giving us ideas, dinner and a movie. Some plays that were going on in town. The Museum of Science was close by as well. Maybe they were trying to tell us something.

When Steve and I had a moment to ourselves that day, I asked him what he would like to do on Saturday.

"I think I would like to take it easy, maybe spend the day at your mother's house. Maybe have the kids come down. Do you think that Marybeth would be able to drive them down?" I could hear in his voice how much he missed them.

"I don't know. I'll call her tonight and find out."

We talked for a while and between the two of us decided that it might not be a good idea for the little ones to see him out of the hospital if he wasn't able to go back home with them. They would never understand why. It was hard enough on them without having them have to deal with that as well.

We were sitting out on the patio. There were tables and chairs and some benches. There were some small gardens built into the wall that some of the patients tended to. The view from the wall was of the Charles River. There was a bridge that was constantly going up to allow the taller boats access to the harbor.

The trains also went by. They were going into and out of North Station. Steve would joke about hopping one and just going home. But he knew it wouldn't be long.

There was only one thing I hated about being out on the patio and that was that you could watch Med Life helicopters landing and rushing patients to the Boston hospitals. I would freeze up inside remembering Steve on that first day and that it was the same route he took to Mass. General. Each time one of them landed I would say a prayer for whoever they were transporting and another one for the family that was on their way to the hospital.

Steve put his arm around me and held me close to him. I couldn't help but think that if it hadn't been for those people that rushed him through the air, he wouldn't be here to comfort me. I thank the good Lord for them.

I was awake at about six o'clock. I stumbled out to the kitchen and started the coffee. My mother had bought a beautiful roast for dinner. She was going to make all of Steve's favorites.

I took a shower, put on my robe and went back out to the kitchen. My mom was up and sitting at the table with a cup of coffee. My thoughts went back to the morning before. My mother and I were sitting at the table over coffee...

&

"Tomorrow when you bring Steve back here, I thought it would be nice if you had some time to yourselves," my Mom said. "It is going to be nice out so I will get your father to take me to a couple of yard sales."

"Ma, you don't have to do that," I said, "Steve just wants a day away from everything. Don't worry about it."

"Laura, I might be older than you, but I'm not that old. I do want you to talk to his doctor though and make sure that," she hesitated, "well that he is strong enough to be left alone with you. Do you understand me?"

She was serious. My mother was arranging for me to have an hour or two alone with my husband. "I'll talk to his doctor, I don't know quite how I'll ask her, but I'll talk to his doctor."

So later in the day before I had left Spaulding, I pulled Dr. Woo aside. "Can I ask you a question, Doctor?"

"Sure, what's up?" She was standing in front of the nurses station. I guided her over to the corridor where we would have more privacy.

"Tomorrow. Well, believe it or not, my mother told me to

talk to you." I was struggling on find a way to talk to her about it.

"Mrs. Merrow, he can do **anything** he wants to do. Anything that he feels he is able to do. Tell your mother not to worry."

ക

...So on Saturday morning I could tell by the look on my mothers' face that she wanted to know if she would be going out with my Dad or not.

"Mom, I talked to his doctor and she said that Steve was fine. That he could do anything he wanted to do. I still think that you shouldn't have to leave. I feel funny."

She told me not to worry about it. She thanked me for 'asking permission' from his doctor, though. She was so concerned about his first day away from the safety of a hospital.

She also wanted to fix everything for him just right. "What time are you planning on getting Steve."

"Well, it's only seven o'clock, I figured we would leave here at about nine or nine thirty, if that's alright with Daddy."

"If what's all right with Daddy?" my father asked as he came into the kitchen. At that moment the phone rang. Daddy picked it up, "Hello?" then he smiled. "Do you mind if I have my coffee first?" Then he handed me the phone. "It's your husband."

I took the phone and smiled "Good morning, how are you feeling?" I asked him.

"I feel great, when are you gonna be here?", exclaimed a very excited Steve.

He sounded very excited. "I just got up Steve, and so did Daddy. What time can you leave?"

"As soon as you get here and I've had my IV."

I asked my father what time he wanted to go. He said as soon as he had his coffee and took a shower. We decided on eight thirty. I told Steve to let me get off the phone so that I could get dressed and drink my coffee.

My Dad and I did what we had to and headed out by about quarter after eight. I'm not sure if Dad was awake or not but he got us there.

Steve was lying on his bed having the last of his IV. His nurse came in and gave me his medications that he would need for the day. She told me that if there were any problems to call her and to get him right back. She smiled and told Steve to have a good day.

Which it was. We went back to the house. We sat and visited for a while before my mother kicked everyone out of the kitchen so she could get dinner ready. Steve and my Dad went out to the porch and played cribbage while my mother and I fixed dinner. I kept wandering out to the porch to see how Steve was doing. We went out to the back yard and sat in the sunshine. I was nervous. I guess that because I didn't have a doctor or a nurse to protect him, and that I was it, made me a little jumpy.

He looked tired, so we went back inside and my Dad put a movie in to watch. Steve stretched out on the couch and I went in to the kitchen to help Mom.

"Is he okay?" my mother asked.

"He's fine. He's just relaxing."

The dinner was delicious. Steve enjoyed every bite of it. Then as my mother had promised, after dinner had been cleared from the table, her and my father went out to hunt for yard sales.

It felt so good to have a day to spend with you with no doctors
or nurses or therapists. Just you and me.

Mom fixed a wonderful dinner. Then her and Dad went out
for a while.

I was so scared. It felt so good having you hold me.
I was shaking. I felt like a girl who knew what was ahead,
but not sure if she would be what he was expecting.

But it was so good. I felt so safe.

I wish I could explain it. For so long I have been trying
to be so strong, trying to protect you. It was so good to
have you hold me and that made me feel safe and protected.

Making love with you today will be a time that will always
be a treasured memory within me. I felt so alive. I felt so
completely loved.

It feels so good to know you will be home soon.

For those couple of hours, the world stood still. The past two months melted away and a love between two people was reborn and rebounded. A living nightmare was washed away by the realization that a love as strong as ours had not died. That we had weathered the storm.

SUNDAY JULY 12, 1992

I was surprised this morning when Steve called me to say that the doctor had released him for the day and that he wanted to spend the day enjoying the outside.

I got dressed and to the hospital as quickly as I could. I think it was about ten o'clock when my Dad dropped me off. The day was beautiful. It was up to about seventy or so and there was a nice warm breeze. The sun was shining. We couldn't have asked for better weather.

We started off by taking a walk to the Science Museum. You could see it from the hospital. It only took about fifteen minutes to get over to it and I'd say about ten of that was trying to cross the main roads.

It was early so it wasn't too crowded. We looked at almost every exhibit. Most of what I watched though was of Steve, though. It was difficult for him to walk around with the patch on one eye and he was very self conscience of it. I'd watch his feet to be sure that he wouldn't trip over anything. I'd watch what was approaching him so that he wouldn't be tripped. I'm sure that I was over doing it and underestimating him, but it couldn't be helped. I was not going to let anything disrupt his progress, nor let anything happen to him that would get in his way of going home.

You could tell that the tour of the museum was taking its toll on him. We stopped and got a cup of coffee and decided to walk over to North Station.

His mother told us of a pizza place that she had gotten a really good sandwich from so we thought we would try to find it and get some lunch. We ended up just ordering a pizza but it was good just the same.

At one point Steve went to the men's room. What only took about two or three minutes seem to take forever to me. I got so anxious that I was going to knock on the door to see if he was okay when the door opened and he emerged. I checked my watch, it was time to start heading back. Marybeth was coming down to visit with the kids this afternoon and I wanted to have Steve back to the hospital in time for his next IV. He didn't want to have to deal with that when the kids were here. He didn't want anything to frighten the little ones this time.

We arrived back to the hospital at about two thirty. By the time the nurse got the IV going it was around three o'clock. Wouldn't you know it, the IV kept slowing down and stopping. What should have only taken ten or fifteen minutes to go through took a total of about forty. By that time, the kids had shown up.

This time the visit was a lot better. Steve was able to sit with the kids. They were a little scared at first but at least this time they reached out their arms and went to him. They talked to him and told him all sorts of stories about events that had happened at home. Becky sat on his lap with her head on his shoulder. The best part was when she looked up and gave him a kiss on the cheek.

Before they left, we brought them down to the cafeteria and treated them all to some frozen yogurt.

We didn't tell them that their Daddy would be home in a few days. As much as we wanted to tell them, it would hurt too much if it didn't happen. Danielle was told though. She was the oldest and the one that was most aware of everything that had happened. I could tell by the look on her face that she had finally heard the one thing that she had waited to hear now for the past two months, Steve and Mom were coming home.

We went to the Science Museum and to lunch.
Walking around Boston with Steve makes me feel so good.
So proud. I want to stop people and say "Hey this is my

husband! Two months ago I wasn't sure if he would live or die. And look! He is here! He is okay! And I am so much in love with him!

The kids were so happy to see him. It did him and them a lot of good.

MONDAY JULY 13, 1992

Today would be a very busy day. They had planned a very aggressive routine in each of his therapy sessions after which we both had a meeting with a Dr. Calvanio. He was the neuro-psychologist at Spaulding and would be giving his recommendation to Dr. Woo as to how he felt Steve would do if released at this time. This doctor already had been through two sessions with Steve and now wanted to have on with me and Steve together.

His schedule for the day started with an outing planned with both occupational therapists and Lynn, the physical therapist. They wanted to see how Steve would do when faced with the public and every day situations. They took us to North Station and the subway. I was told I could go as long as I didn't give him any help. They told me they would terminate the session if I tried to assist or interfere with it in any way.

They asked him to locate different stores at which he had to find out the cost of different items. He had to determine the arrival and departure times of certain trains. Then they took him on to the subway and had him tell us which one to take to get to the Aquarium.

I thought he did fine. His only difficulty was his footing because of the patch. He would be extra cautious going down a flight of stairs or when walking down a very busy sidewalk. The therapists however thought it was because of hidden difficulty. I told them they were wrong. All in all I believe they thought he did fine but that he had to have more confidence in himself. I was sure they would write a good review.

We all walked back together, rather quickly too. I might

add. I think he simply wanted to impress the hell out of them. Personally, I had trouble keeping up with him.

When we got back, Steve and I had just enough time to grab a cup of coffee before heading up to Dr. Calvanio's office. This doctor made me nervous. Steve was very intimidated by him. He felt as though he was the one obstacle between staying here and going home on Wednesday.

Had a meeting with Doctor Calvanio this afternoon. He seems really nice. I realized that there was still lot about everything that you still don't know or understand.

Today we both found out that where the aneurysm had been leaking for so long that slowly different parts of the brain were being affected. Lack of oxygen and insufficient blood flow causes deterioration and it will take a long time for them to rejuvenate.

But by simply hearing this one piece of information triggered something in you. Your need to know and to understand what has happened to you has now surfaced.

I told you some of it but your reaction to the little bit that I did tell you was so strong that I thought it best to tell you the whole thing once I had you back home.

When we finished with Dr. Calvanio we went back to your room. As you went in to see if your dinner had arrived I noticed Dr. Woo discussing something with Lynn, the physical therapist. I wandered down to where they were standing.

"Hello Mrs. Merrow. I hope your time with Dr. Calvanio was productive." Dr. Woo always seemed to be so cheerful. She never pulled punches with me though.

I only had one question to ask her. "Can you tell me whether or not you are going to release Steve for Wednesday?"

"We were just discussing your outing." She looked at Lynn

and then back to me. "His therapy has gone well and I don't think there is very much more that we can offer him here."

Lynn interrupted her, "I have recommended an extended program for him though. It is called 'work hardening' and is offered by some rehabilitation hospitals. I think it will do him a lot of good."

"Not only that, Mrs. Merrow," Dr. Woo added, "but his speech therapist thinks that he may need an additional outpatient therapy session set up after he is released."

I shook my head, "I can understand the work hardening, but I don't fully agree with the other. I've sat in on all the sessions with Steve and some of the tests he has been given even I couldn't understand them. Aside from that, the insurance I had when Steve was admitted here has been cancelled and I doubt seriously that it will be extended to cover an outpatient program of any kind."

Dr. Woo nodded, "I'll keep that in mind and make a few phone calls. I'll have some answers for you by tomorrow. As far as him being able to go home on Wednesday," she smiled and took my hands, "he's all yours!"

My heart felt as though it was standing still. Two more days. In two more days, this entire nightmare would come to an end.

"Thank you." It came out as a whisper. "Thank you so much, for everything."

I turned and walked back to Steve's room. He was sitting on the edge of the bed eating his dinner. "I hope you don't mind me eating in front of you, princess, but I am starving." He barely looked up from his plate.

"No that's all right." I sat down on the bed next to him. My heart was back to life and beating a mile a minute.

He gulped down his milk and asked, "What were you talking to the doctor about? Anything good?"

"Well, let me say this, tomorrow after your therapy sessions I guess I could help you pack up all this garbage and get you ready to go home on Wednesday."

"Really?" He put his arms around me. "I'm going home. I'm

really going home." He held me for about five or ten minutes. I didn't say anything, but I knew he just didn't want me to see his face. He was crying.

He didn't want me to tell anybody. He didn't want to jinx it in any way. I didn't know if I could do that. I would have to tell my parents. I was going to have to tell Marybeth. She was the one who was coming to get us and bring us home. He knew better, by the end of the night everyone and their uncles would know. It was about time that I had good news to share.

TUESDAY JULY 14, 1992

Finished up your therapy sessions today.

Dr. Woo feels it will be okay for you to go home and not worry about therapy for a while. She said to come back and see her in a month.

I am so scared about tomorrow. I get nervous that you will wake up and have a fever.

I wish that it was all over right now. That I was curled up in
your arms and feeling safe and warm.

Please dear God, let it be okay. Let it be over.

Although Dr. Woo signed his release to go home she sat and talked to me about what I was facing once Steve got home. She told me to watch for violent mood swings. That it could be a sign of something wrong. To be sure that he kept up with his exercising that Lynn had taught him.

Most of all she told me that she wanted me to continue with the support. She had been so impressed with the fact that I showed up every morning and stayed till the end of the day. She had not seen too many spouses play such an active role in the recovery process.

I told her that I had to be here. That I had been with Steve every step of the way. How could I possibly support his recovery if I had not participated in it from the start? I could not fathom how I could have handled it differently. I had no idea how anybody else could not be here with their spouse. Though I had seen it. Patients sitting alone day after day. It was so sad.

She said that a lot of people could not or would not know how to handle it. That seeing someone they love in a state that they could not function in the way that they used to was a hard thing to deal with. But she knew that Steve would be okay. We were both bound and determined to see this through until the end.

The rest of the day seemed to take so long to pass by us. As hard as we tried to not talk about it, the fact that he was going home the next day was ever present in our hearts. We were almost afraid to say anything out loud for fear that something would happen. Perhaps if we said it aloud, the magical bubble would burst and we wouldn't be able to leave.

A nurse would take his temperature and I'd wait to hear what it was. At four o'clock it rose to about ninety nine. I must have gone white. Steve just looked at me and reminded me that every day his temp went up a little about this time.

I told him that I needed to go back to my mother's and that I would call him later. I gave him a hug and a kiss. It was so hard to leave.

By the time I got back to my parents house and had eaten supper there was a knock on the door. It was Marybeth.

"Thought you might want some company," she said. She was such a good friend. We sat and talked for a while and made sure of the time she would be here in the morning to get Steve.

"Get your shoes on, we're going out," she said.

I hesitated, but she told me I need to get out and to stop thinking about everything and to get away from the phone.

"I told Steve that I would call him later though." I wasn't sure what to do.

She smiled, "So call him now," she said, "Call him and tell him we are going out to eat."

So I did. I told him we wouldn't be out long and I would call him when we got back.

We went down the street to a little place that my sister Debby waitresses at. Marybeth bought me a drink and we talked. She knew how nervous I was and told me to ease up. That I needed to calm down.

"I'm just so afraid that something is going to go wrong. I don't think he can handle it if something stops him from leaving tomorrow."

"Nothing is going to happen." She ordered me one more drink and when it was gone, I told her it was time to leave.

It had been raining really hard before we left. Outside Marybeth told me I was too uptight. Before I knew it she had stomped her foot into a huge puddle and got me good. I was drenched from my feet to my waist. All I could do was laugh. It felt really good. I stomped my foot into the same puddle to try and get her wet too, but as hard as I tried I couldn't aim well enough to get her. Each puddle she found though had my name on it. I laughed all the way back to my parent's house. I was soaked from head to toe by the time we got back.

We walked into my parent's kitchen as quietly as we could. My dad heard us and came to see if we were all right. When he saw me trying to peel the socks off of my feet and saw how wet we were, he just chuckled. He opened the hall closet and tossed us each a towel. Then chuckled again and went back to the living room.

Marybeth was right. I did need to calm down a little. It felt so good to laugh again. It seemed like so long ago that I heard that noise coming out of my mouth.

Marybeth left, promising to be there as early as she could. She said her father was letting us use his car. It would be more comfortable for Steve than using her truck, or risking my car. The two of us had planned at one point to get Steve a limo, but without knowing exactly what day we would need it, and after the scare at Mass General we chose to forget that idea. She told me that her father's car was nice and roomy and Steve would be very comfortable in it for the ride home.

I gave her a hug and thanked her for everything. She had been so patient with me and so helpful throughout this whole thing.

"Hey, it was not a problem," she smiled, gave me a hug and went on her way.

WEDNESDAY JULY 15, 1992

I was awakened by the phone ringing. I bolted out of bed and rushed to pick it up. I looked at the clock. It was a quarter to seven.

"Hello?"

"Good morning, darlin'!" It was Steve.

"What's wrong?" My heart was in my throat.

"Nothing. I just called to say good morning and to find out what time you were going to be here."

"Oh, are you sure you are okay? What's your temp this morning? Have the nurses come in yet?"

He laughed a little, "Will you chill out? I am okay, and my temp is fine. The nurse was in a little while ago."

My mother was coming out of her bedroom, "Is that Steve?"

"Yes, Mom" I reached for a cigarette and the lighter. As I lit it my hands were shaking.

"Is everything all right?" she asked.

"Yes Mom, he is only calling to say good morning." I turned my conversation back to Steve. "Marybeth will be here at about nine o'clock and we will probably be there no later than ten o'clock." -

I finished my conversation with Steve, got off of the phone and joined my mother at the kitchen table. She got up and poured me a cup of coffee and then sat with me. "Is he all set to go home this morning?"

I laughed. "He is chomping at the bit. I think if he had his way he would have had Marybeth and I sleep in the car in the parking lot!"

"What about you?" my mother asked, "Do you have all your things ready?"

"Yes, Marybeth and I put a lot of it in her truck last night and the rest is packed. I did all that before I went to bed last night."

As I drank my coffee it started to sink in that today was it. Today I would finally be taking my husband home.

My mother got ready for work and we said our good byes. It was hard. We both held back the tears. We had been through hell and back together and now it was over. I tried to thank her but it wasn't enough. All I could do was hug her and tell her how grateful I was that I had her and Daddy there to lean on. I didn't know what I would have done without them.

I watched her leave and started to cry. I brushed the tears away. I didn't have time for this. I had to shower and get dressed. I put on a fresh pot of coffee and hopped into the shower.

When I got out I called Steve.

"Hi!" I said when he answered the phone.

"Hi again. What are you doing? Is Marybeth there yet?" he asked.

"No, I just wanted to call and see how you were. I wasn't awake before. Did I already ask you if the nurse was in yet?"

"I wish you would stop asking me that" he replied. "I am fine but your are going to jinx me if you don't stop checking on me."

We talked for a minute before I realized that Marybeth would be here and I was still in my robe. I got off of the phone and hurried to get dressed. I had laid out a skirt and a pink top. I wanted to look nice for him.

I must have brushed my hair a dozen times and checked my makeup just as many. I couldn't believe how nervous I was.

I kept looking at the clock. Eight forty five. Nine o'clock. Nine fifteen. Nine thirty. Where was she? I tried to call her and her father answered the phone.

"Hi Mr. White, this is Lauri Merrow. Marybeth still isn't there is she?"

"No..." he hesitated. "She left almost an hour ago. She really should be there by now." He sounded very concerned.

"Oh okay. I'm sure she'll be here any minute. She probably got stuck in traffic." I didn't want to sound too concerned myself. I knew that she was driving his car and I didn't want to upset him.

"Well, do me a favor, will you?" he asked. "When she gets there have her call me. She's never driven my car. As a matter of fact I've hardly driven it that much. It's new you know."

No, I didn't know that. Marybeth hadn't told me that the car she was borrowing was a brand new one. "I'm sure everything is fine, Mr. White, but I will have her call you." As I hung up the receiver I could hear a car pulling up out front. It was her. She laughed when I told her that she was going to have to call her father. As she did and was on the phone with him, I loaded the last of my bags into the trunk of the car. A few minutes later we were on our way to Spaulding.

The sky was overcast and there was a slight mist in the air. I took it as a good sign. It had been cloudy and miserable the day he went in. It only seemed fitting that it was the same type of day on his way home.

When we arrived at the hospital he was all set and ready to go. I looked for his nurse and when I found her she seemed surprised with my question.

"When will Dr. Woo be here to sign him out?" I asked.

"Oh the doctor already signed his release form, he can leave any time he wants." She handed me the prescriptions for his tegritol and gave me enough to carry him over to the end of the day in case we didn't get if filled until tomorrow.

I just stood there. I felt as though I should be waiting for the doctor. So didn't Steve and Marybeth. It just didn't feel right to leave without someone having something signed.

I asked the nurse, "Don't we have to sign something saying that he is being released?"

"No, he is all set," and she walked away.

That was it?

We grabbed his suitcase, his balloons and the rest of his things and called for the elevator. We all felt the same way. It felt so great and exhilarating leaving, but we all kept looking over our shoulders half expecting someone to stop us. It was almost as though we were helping him to escape.

But nobody stopped us. We put his things in the trunk. Steve sat up front with Marybeth and I climbed in back. Steve and Marybeth started talking and my thoughts went over everything that had happened. It took about five minutes for it to sink into me. We were on our way home. I wouldn't have to come back here again. It was over. A tear fell down my cheek. Then another, and another. I silently wept and told the Lord thank you for His help. Steve turned around and smiled. He knew. He reached back and took my hand. He held onto it for most of the ride home.

Home. I could hardly believe it was true. We were finally on our way home. I looked in my bag beside me. My journals were tucked inside. They were closed now. Hopefully, I wouldn't have to add to them.

THE DAYS AT HOME....

So many people, so many times had warned me that I should be prepared for a lot of work, a lot of uphill climbing once I got Steve home. I had always put it in the back of my mind and concentrated more on the road I had been on, getting Steve back on his feet and bring him home.

I should have listened. I was not prepared for the roller coaster ride that I was suddenly put on. The first few days home were very predictable. Steve spent a lot of time in bed, resting and taking special moments to get back into his children's lives.

He was so careful to be sure that he took his medicine on time, never to miss a pill. The fear of having a seizure was ever present to both of us.

He was faithful to his exercise regime. The two of us would go through the routine each day and take turns on the exercise bike.

He took hold of each day and did his utmost to take care of himself. He was nervous, and so was I. He would lie down to rest, or to take a nap, and I would tiptoe to the bedroom just to make sure he was okay. He always was.

It would take a few days for me to be able to sleep through an entire night. I felt so safe being next to him, feeling him hold me, but I was afraid to fall asleep. I would lie there and listen to him breathe.

I found out two days after Steve had come home, that Linda Grant had to be operated on. She needed a hip replacement and would be up at the hospital only a couple of blocks away. The day of the surgery came and she pulled through with flying colors. The next morning, I called her hospital room.

"I'm okay....," her voice trailed. She was heavily medicated.

"I'll be up soon to see you." I hung up the phone. I was so relieved to know that she was all right. I got a sick feeling in the pit of my stomach at the thought of going up to see her. I cringed at the thought of going into another hospital. I felt so guilty. She had been so good to me. No one had done as much for me during the past two months as she had. Yet I was terrified to go into the hospital to visit her.

The next morning, the phone rang. It was Linda. She was a bit more coherent this time. "When are you coming to see me?"

"I'll be there soon." I didn't know what to say to her.

"If you are not coming, just say so. I thought we were friends." She sounded so disappointed.

"I want to see you, but I just don't know if I can bring myself to walk into the hospital. I don't know how to explain it. I don't want to hurt you. I'm just scared, I don't know how to put it into words. I hope you understand."

"No, I don't. I am okay. I just need you to be here."

I got off the phone and went into the bedroom. Steve followed me. "What's wrong?" he asked.

I told him. He came over and sat with me for a minute. "Do what you want, I'll go up to see her tonight. Marybeth will be here, she'll go with me. But Linda is your best friend. She needs you. If it was the other way around she'd be there for you." At that comment he turned and walked out of the room.'

I started to sob violently, almost hysterically. I felt so alone. Why couldn't they understand?

By the time Marybeth showed up I had pulled myself together and decided to go. I made them promise that we would only stay for a little while.

We walked over and up to the second floor to her room. My throat tightened. I don't know why, but I wanted to run. I didn't, but I didn't want to be there either.

She was asleep. I went to the side of her bed and took her hand. My mind flashed to the night of Steve's surgery, and the moment I took his hand and felt him try to hold it. Linda opened her eyes. "You're here. I'm okay," her voice was just above a whisper. "They just gave me something for pain, so I'm really groggy..."

Her eyes focused on Steve. "Hey, you're here too. You look great." She saw Marybeth and thanked them for coming to visit.

The three of them talked. The entire time she held onto my hand. Before we left I bent down and gave her a kiss on the forehead. "I'll be back to see you in a few days." I wasn't sure if I could do it, but I would try.

All I wanted to do was forget about hospitals, about people in pain, about everything.

A week after Steve came home, I went onto unemployment benefits and realized that we were financially okay. Between his disability benefits and my unemployment pay we would be all right.

We spent each day enjoying the kids, exercising and taking advantage of each day. We took the kids to the lake when it was warm enough on the weekends.

Steve wouldn't swim, though. He would wade out to about his waist and then come back to the shore and sit with me. When I asked him why, he told me he wasn't sure if he remembered how to swim. He said he felt as though everyone was watching him. I told him it would come in time. A lot of things would. We both needed to be patient. For now, we just needed to be together.

We had planned a huge party for the labor day weekend. It was a double celebration. Becky was turning two and we wanted to celebrate Steve being home.

So everybody that helped him pull through was invited to the party. My parents, his mother, his sisters, my sisters and all of our nieces and nephews. Sue, Marybeth, and Linda Grant and her family. We also invited his Aunt Bev and Uncle Leo.

It was wonderful. Becky was showered with birthday gifts and Steve was showered with gifts as well. Everyone was in awe over the fact that he was there to celebrate. It was a wonderful time. It left me with a feeling of relief.

Maybe it was over. Maybe now we could relax. Maybe.....

SATURDAY SEPTEMBER 5, 1992

I was woken by a loud crash. I looked at the clock. It was five thirty in the morning. I reached my arm out for Steve, the other half of the bed was empty. I must have heard the bathroom door shutting. I rolled over and fell back to sleep. A little while later, about twenty minutes or so, I was awoken again. This time it was the bathroom door and Steve was coming back into the bedroom.

I took one look at him and my heart stood still. His face was as white as a sheet and he had beads of sweat pouring down his forehead.

"What's wrong?"

"Lauri, I am really sick. I don't feel well at all." He was at the end of the bed and crawled up to his pillow. He was trembling, and shaking all over. I felt his forehead. It was a little warm, but not so much as to be feverish.

"What happened?" I asked him. I pulled the blanket up over him.

"I don't know," he started, "I remember getting up to go to the bathroom. I went out to the kitchen to get a smoke and felt really dizzy. So I laid down on the floor and the next thing I knew I woke up and was soaking wet. I must have gotten a drink of water and spilt it." He was shivering, so I tried tucking the blankets tight around him.

I didn't know what to do. "Are you having a headache?"

"No, I just feel as weak as a kitten. Let me lie here for a few minutes and I'll let you know how I feel."

I got up to get myself a cigarette and to see how much water had spilt onto the floor. The floor was soaked. I grabbed a towel and got down on the floor to wipe the mess. The smell that hit me was unmistakable. This wasn't water on the floor, it was urine. And a lot of it. I mopped it up and put the towels in a pail to be washed. As I was walking back towards the bedroom, I stepped on something. A cigarette butt. There was also a burn mark on the floor. This must have been Steve's cigarette. If Steve had dropped a cigarette, he never would have left it. That is of course if he knew he had dropped it. Something wasn't right. He couldn't have just lied down because he felt dizzy. I ran back into the bedroom.

"What happened to you?" I asked.

He looked puzzled. "What do you mean?"

"I mean what happened in the kitchen? Did you lie down or did you fall down? And it wasn't water that spilt on the floor. I just mopped up a floor covered with your urine. Now tell me what happened?" My voice was rising. I was getting scared.

He looked scared too. "I told you," he said, "I felt dizzy and lied down. I didn't think I could make it back to the bedroom, so I lied down on the floor. I told you I had gotten up to go to the bathroom, maybe I fainted or fell asleep and pissed. I don't know. I'm sorry you had to clean it up." He looked at me with a fright in his eyes. "You think I had a seizure, don't you. I didn't. I would have known. I simply lied down."

I wasn't sure. If he had gone through even a mild seizure, he wouldn't remember. I didn't know what to think. I knew that something was wrong though. I went back out to the kitchen to light a cigarette, that's when I noticed the cabinet doors. They were all open. All the doors near where I had found the cigarette butt were open. Why? Maybe that was the crash I heard.

I could hear footsteps from behind me. I turned around and saw Jimmy standing there. "Is Steve okay?" he asked.

"Why? Did you hear something?" I saw a look of major concern and fright on his face.

"Well, I heard this big bang, then I heard somebody moaning. It sounded like Steve. I was too scared to come and see."

"He's in bed, honey. I think he fell. Don't worry. He's okay."

I sent him into the living room to watch cartoons. That did it for me though. As much as Steve denied it, I felt that he had gone through some type of seizure. I didn't push it with him though.

I asked him if I should call the doctor at Mass General. He told me to wait and see if he felt any better after a little bit more sleep. I didn't want to wait, but I did. For about half an hour.

I peeked back in on him. He was still wide awake and still shivering. I got the thermometer and took his temperature. It was about ninety nine point five. It wasn't too high, but it still bothered me. This time I didn't ask. "I'm calling your doctor."

"If you do," he said, "he is going to tell you to bring me in to the hospital." He looked at me with the look of a frightened child. "I don't want to go back."

"I'm calling. You're shaking like a leaf and Jim says he heard you moaning last night. Something is wrong. I want to find out what it is. Maybe it's nothing. Maybe I'm being over protective. Laugh at me later and tell me 'I told you so'. But right now, I am calling Dr. Ogilvy."

I went out to the kitchen and dialed his number. He was not on call but Dr. Crowell would return my call, I was told by the answering service. So I paced.

About ten minutes later the telephone rang. It was Doctor Crowell. I told him what I knew and he told me what I knew he would. Get him to Mass General. He would notify the emergency room that we were coming in.

I called Marybeth. I told her what was going on and asked her if she would come over and watch the kids while I brought him in. As always, Marybeth was there for me. No problem, she told me.

Steve was in the emergency room about two hours later. Doctor Yu looked at him. They took him for a cat scan and then we waited.

Finally after what seemed like hours, Doctor Yu came back to tell us the results. "There seems to be some swelling in the ventricals. This would mean that the shunt is not draining the CSF properly. That is the cerebral..."

I cut him off. "I know what CSF is. What now? What happens now??"

"Well, we'll have to see where the shunt is blocked and unblock it." He made it sound so simple. He took out a needle and explained that he was going to insert it into the top of the shunt. He told us that it was common for this to happen and that this should do the trick.

I watched as he inserted the needle through Steve's scalp into the part of the shunt that caused a large bump on the top of his head.

He drew back on the needle and tried to flush the fluid back through. I could tell by the frown on his face that it didn't work the way he wanted it to. He tried a couple of more times. Each time with a new needle.

Finally he said that he was going to call Dr. Schumaker and see if he had any thoughts. He told us not to worry.

About five minutes later I saw him on the phone. I was too far away to pick up the entire conversation but I did hear him the person he was talking to, probably Dr. Schumaker, that he had done that already.

When he was off the phone he came over to us and told us that Dr. Schumaker was on his way over to see if he could flush it.

Well, Dr. Schumaker did the same thing that Dr. Yu had tried. It worked just as well as it had the first time around. Steve said that he could feel the needles crackling inside his head. He said he wasn't in any pain, but that he could feel the pressure of them trying to flush it through.

Dr. Schumaker decided that he wanted Steve to spend the night at the hospital. He said that sometimes after trying to flush it unsuccessfully that the next day it would work.

Steve however, had different ideas. "Well, then can I go home and come back tomorrow?" He gave them a brilliant case, but Dr. Schumaker stood fast.

Steve was admitted for overnight observation and would hopefully go home the next day.

By the end of the day Steve was settled in a room on the

twelfth floor. Back in the Ellison Building. The same place he had been before, with the same nurses on duty. Leann had been assigned to him. I felt as though I had been thrown back in time, back into a nightmare that seemed to have no end.

SUNDAY SEPTEMBER 6, 1992

I had called Marybeth from the hospital yesterday and told her what was going on. She agreed with me and Dr. Schumaker, Steve should stay. I asked her if she would mind spending the night with the kids. As always, no problem. She asked me if I called my parents. I told her that I had tried but that I was going to have to call them back, my mother had been on the phone.

Well, I guess my mother had returned my call not knowing where I had called from and Marybeth had filled her in a little. I called my mother as soon as our conversation ended.

"Do you want us to come in?" my mother asked.

"No, I'm just waiting for Steve to be settled in and if it's okay I'd like to spend the night at your house."

She told me that it was fine but that I should have called them earlier so that I wouldn't have had to go through this all by myself.

"Mom, I'm not alone. Steve's here. I've been in the emergency room with him anyway. You and Daddy would have been in the waiting room by yourselves. Besides, we didn't know what was going on."

So here I was back at my parents house the following day. I was making coffee and trying to wake up. I looked at the clock. Seven thirty. The nurses should be changing shifts, maybe Leann was on duty.

I wanted to talk to the nurses before I talked to Steve. Something seemed to be gnawing at me and I felt very odd. I didn't know what it was.

I sat down and called the nurses station. Good, Leann was there.

"Hi Mrs. Merrow. This is Leann," she was quiet.

"Hi Leann, how's my husband this morning?" I asked.

"His fever is up a little." She had a hesitation to her voice. "They brought him down for another cat scan."

"Another one? They just did one yesterday." I started to get scared again. "What's going on?"

"I'm not sure," she said, "They think there may be an infection in the shunt. If there is they will have to replace it. Are you coming in this morning?"

"I'll be there in half an hour."

"Take your time, they just brought him down for the cat scan, he won't be back up for about another forty minutes."

"I'll be there in half an hour," I repeated and hung up the phone.

Leann had misjudged the time. By the time I got to the hospital they had just brought Steve back to his room. He was covered with three blankets and was shivering.

Leann came into the room. "I tried to call you, but you had just left. I'm glad you're here."

"What's happened? What's wrong with him?" I looked from her to him and back again. I was panic stricken.

"There is an infection. They just put him in for an emergency surgery to replace the shunt. Dr. Schumaker is going to do it." She told us that Steve was on call for the next available operating room.

I was in a daze. I couldn't believe this was happening. I sat down on the bed next to him. I rubbed his back and his arms in the hopes that it might help him to get warmer.

He was so pale. He understood what she had told us. He didn't seem to care so long as he could feel better.

It couldn't have been more that five or ten minutes later when an orderly followed by Leann came into the room.

"It's time to go Steve," Leann called out.

They put him on the gurney and wheeled him away. I

turned to the window and started to cry. Leann came up behind me and put her hands on my shoulders.

"I'm sorry," I said to her. "I just can't believe this is happening."

"I know, neither can I." she replied. "You can stay in here and wait for him and if you do leave the floor I will find you when it's over. It should only take an hour or two once they get started."

"I want to talk to Dr. Schumaker when it's over. Tell him that. Don't let him leave the floor until I can talk to him, please."

I sat down and started to make the phone calls. First on the list was my mom. She told me that she would call everybody else for me and that my father was on his way up to stay with me. She was something else. Right there for me as always. I was so grateful to her for making my calls. I didn't know how to do it this time. I knew that everybody else had the same feeling as I did just a week ago. That maybe we could relax. That maybe our fears were going to fade away.

I couldn't tell them that there were more reasons to be afraid.

The wait was just as hard this time as it was before. My Dad took me down to Brigham's for lunch and we talked.

When we got back to Steve's room Leann was waiting for us.

"I just got off the phone with Dr. Schumaker. You have great timing." She reached into her pocket and pulled out a piece of paper. "I wrote it down as best as I could remember. I know you kept everything in a notebook. Dr. Schumaker said that he is fine and that they could not replace the shunt yet."

"What? Why not?" I sat down. "What went wrong this time?"

"Well let me read what I wrote, 'There was infection in both the brain and in the stomach. That it was real screwy.'" She shook her head. "They had to do another ventriculostomy. We will keep him on antibiotics for a while and then they will put the new shunt in once the infection clears up."

I let it all sink in. She gave me her note to keep and told me that Dr. Schumaker wanted us to wait for him in Steve's room and that he would be up shortly to talk to us.

Leann went back to her duties and my father came over to me and put his arm around my shoulders and pulled me to him. "He's going to be just fine," he said.

A short while later the doctor came in to tell us what had happened. He was almost bouncing with excitement. "I am so amazed with your husband! He has cheated death one more time."

At that moment he composed himself realizing how upset I was and apologized. "It's just that I am so happy with everything. The tubing for the shunt was so severely infected that the infection just pushed it right out of him. It was like a snake when it did that." He was motioning at his neck as if to make a clearer picture of what he was trying to tell me. "However, because of the infection we had to just take the whole thing out. We'll put it back in a few days. Let the antibiotics take care of the infection." He put his hand on my shoulder, "You okay?" he asked. "He is in recovery and will be up in an hour or so. Don't worry, he's just fine. He's one hell of a guy. Our own little miracle man. I'll be in touch." At that, he turned on his heel and was on his way.

One thing that he said stood fast in my mind. "Your husband has cheated death again!" My God, what had happened? What if I had listened to Steve and hadn't brought him in when I did? What if he had gotten his way and went home last night? I almost lost him again. Whatever had happened could have killed him...again.

My father pulled me to him, "The doctor said he was okay." There were tears in his eyes. "He'll be fine. He's a stubborn man. He'll be fine," he said. I put my head on his shoulder and cried.

We both were probably thinking the same thing. Why? But most of all, we were relieved to know that he HAD cheated death again. We still had him with us.

I felt as though somebody had held the world still. My father guided me to the elevator and we went out to the courtyard for a cigarette.

Afterward, I called Marybeth, my mom and Steve's family. I couldn't bring myself to tell them all how close he had come. In a way, if I didn't speak of it, then maybe it hadn't happened.

While I talked to his sister, she mentioned her baby's baptism. Steve was the God-father. She told me that she had postponed it. It was scheduled for next week. Not only was Steve the God-father but I was supposed to sing. It was now on for the twenty seventh. I told her I wasn't sure if Steve would be able to be there, but that I would still sing her song. It was a song that I had written the music to of a poem that she wrote.

She understood. We didn't know if Steve would be in the hospital or not on that date. Even if he was home, whether or not he would be up to attending.

Her main concern and prayers were for her brother. I told

her that everything would be okay. Deep in my heart however, I really wasn't sure. For me too, the only thing I could do was pray.

This time everything went differently. I had my car, so I didn't have to take the subway. Steve was able to speak for himself, so doctors were not consulting with me every step of the way. But the biggest change was that I wasn't able to stay with him every day. The kids were starting school on Wednesday and need me home. This was Dawn's very first day of school and it would be hard enough on her having Steve in the hospital again, but I couldn't let her face that day without me as well.

So I would spend most of Monday with Steve and head back to Methuen on Tuesday. It tore me apart to leave him, but the kids needed me more. I had to go home. The nurses and doctors would take care of Steve but there would be not replacing Dawn's first day of school.

It was really upsetting to Steve having to be there on that day too. He told me that he had missed so much this year and now he was going to miss yet another important event. He insisted that I go home which made it a little easier. I promised him that I would take a lot of pictures. Which I did. From the bath the night before, to cookies and milk after school. We got pictures of Dawn in the school yard, with her kindergarten teacher all the way to getting off of the bus for the very first time.

After her snack, I let Dawn call her Daddy at the hospital and tell him all about her day. We took pictures of that too.

We all spent a lot of time on the phone with Steve. I would ask him all sorts of questions that I wasn't able to ask the doctors this time around.

According to what I had been told, the ventricular drain was only to stay there for a few days and then they would put the new shunt in. They kept putting it off. They wanted to be extremely careful that the infection had been completely taken care of.

By Thursday Steve was climbing the walls. He couldn't understand why they just didn't do the surgery and put in the new shunt. I, myself, was fairly content that they hadn't. I hoped that they would wait until the weekend so that I could be at the hospital.

Friday afternoon I packed some of my things and headed back to Boston. Marybeth would be staying with the kids for the weekend.

I don't know what I would have done this time without her. She was right there for me. She gave up her weekends without question. Without her and Linda Grant to help me, I don't know what I would have done.

I go to Boston before the rush hour traffic had begun. It couldn't have been any later than two or three o'clock. Before I could go up to Steve's room, I had to stop in at the financial aid department. We didn't have any insurance this time and a woman had called me yesterday about filling out forms for hospital free care. She told me to gather all of Steve's W-2 forms as well as mine and to stop into her office this afternoon.

She was a very nice woman. She took down all the information and told me not to worry, that we qualified for the free care program and the last thing I should have on my mind was the cost of his care.

The entire process was going to take some time, and we wouldn't be getting forms to sign until once Steve had been sent home. I sat with her for close to an hour before we were finished.

By the time I got upstairs it was about three thirty. Steve's mother and her friend Tom were there. They had brought Steve some goodies he told me. He reached over to his bedside table and opened the drawer. It was filled with chocolates, mints, gum and magazines. He told me that they weren't all from Tom and his mother, but that my parents had been by as well the night before and had given him some of it. I laughed. There was enough sugar in the drawer to turn him into a diabetic.

We went down to the lounge to visit. Steve wasn't able

to go outdoors because of the fear that he would get a further infection.

After his Mom and Tom left. Steve and I spent some time alone. He was scared. He was so aware of what was going on this time. I didn't know what to say to him other than he would pull through this time just as well if not better than the time before. That compared to the last time he was here, this was a piece of cake.

It wasn't much comfort to him though. What worsened his fear was his anxiety over when they would get the new shunt put in. We were told that it would not be done this weekend, but would be done early in the week. Steve was furious.

He told me that other that the fact that he had a tube coming out of his head, that he felt fine and that it was not fair for him to have to wait.

Aside from all of that he had a rather loud roommate. He was a young man, no more that twenty-five. His family seemed to be born again Christians. They would be in the room preaching until eleven or twelve o'clock at night. If not them, then his wife would be there with their two young children. A little girl no more than four years old and an infant about six weeks old. When they left it only got worse. Steve told me that his roommate snored extremely loud all night. I guess that a nurse once offered Steve a sleeping pill it was so bad. But Steve wouldn't take it. He hated stuff like that.

Steve just suffered through it all in the hopes that they would do his surgery and let him go home.

The weekend seemed to fly. It was Sunday afternoon before I knew it and I had to leave. No word of exactly when they would operate other than "early part of the week". That and if all went well with the surgery, Steve would be able to go home a few days after that.

Steve told me that he didn't want me to feel that I had to be there for the surgery. I could worry and pace at home. He was worried about our car dying. It was on its last legs and I would need it to get him home with.

I kissed him good-bye and headed home by three o'clock

in order to avoid the traffic. Halfway home the tears started streaming down my face. I wasn't sure why I was crying. I was so tired and drained. I was terrified that this nightmare would go on and on forever. I desperately needed someone to take care of me. I felt so selfish feeling this way, but it seemed that I was being pulled apart and I just didn't know how to hold myself together anymore. How I longed for someone to tell me that it was okay. For somebody to tell me that I was not crazy.

I pulled myself together by the time I got home. I looked at Marybeth and she knew. I asked her if she could stay for a little while.

She helped me get supper and then helped me get the kids to bed. She told me to sit down and she brought me a glass of wine. "I know you don't drink anymore, but you need to chill out," she placed it in from of me and told me to drink it.

"I know that he is going to be fine. I just don't know if I will survive this. I feel like I am cracking up. I feel so damn alone."

"Listen, it's okay. You've been through hell and back. Nobody has done more than you have. What you really need is a vacation."

"What I really need is my Steve." I picked up the phone and called him. It was a short conversation, but I needed to know he was okay. After I got off the phone Marybeth told me that I worry too much.

It seemed like that was all I knew how to do. All that was left for me to do.

WEDNESDAY SEPTEMBER 16, 1992

Steve called me mid-morning. "They are going to do it!" His voice was both excited and nervous.

"Are they sure, they said it would definitely be today?" I prayed that they would stick to their decision. They told him the same thing yesterday and then put it off until today.

"Yup, I am 'on call'. Leann just came in and told me."

"God, I hope so." I knew what the answer would be, but I asked just the same, "Are you sure you don't want me there? I know I can work something out with somebody."

He was firm in his reply. "No honey, I'll need you more by the weekend. I'd rather you saved the babysitters for then. I'll be okay." Then as an afterthought, "I am nervous but at least this time I can talk on the phone to you."

And talk we did, I called him about once every hour to see if they had confirmed a time yet. I knew from past experience that being on call with them meant that when they were ready for you there was not much notice.

I called his nurse, Leann, and told her to call me when they brought him down. She told me it would probably be around five or six o'clock, but she wasn't sure. She also said that they could be running ahead of schedule and take him sooner. I made sure she had my phone number and told her to call me as soon as he went down and that I wanted Dr. Schumaker, who would be the attending surgeon, to call me when it was over.

I was surprised that I didn't wear a path in the floor. I paced all afternoon. Finally at about four-thirty or so the phone rang.

"They are getting me ready to do down. I should be going in about twenty minutes or so."

"I love you Steve," I swallowed back the tears, "I wish I could be there with you."

"I love you too, princess," he said, "Don't worry, I know you want to be here. You are...in spirit. In my heart."

That was the understatement of the century. I couldn't think of anything else. About twenty-five minutes later, I got a call from his nurse telling me that they just took him. It would be about an hour or so before anything started because they had to prep him. I looked up at the clock, that would make it about six-thirty on the outside that they would start. I made sure she remembered to have the doctor call me when it was all over. She said that she wrote it down in his chart so that the doctor would be sure to see it.

I don't know how I functioned, but I managed to get the supper on the table and feed everyone. While I was clearing the table there was a tap on the door and in walked Marybeth.

A sigh came through me, "You don't know how good your timing is." I told her what was going on, "I haven't even called anybody yet."

"I told you before, you should not have to be calling everybody, they should be calling you." She started a pot of water for tea. "Listen, this is hard enough on you as it is, you should not have to worry about who you have to make phone calls to."

I shook my head, "I know what you're saying, but nobody knows that he is in surgery."

"I know, but still, they knew it would be sometime today. Why put yourself through that? Let them call you."

She was right. Each time I called somebody, I had to relive each detail all over again. Even still, I made the phone calls. I had to.

When I was done, we put the kids to bed and sat down in the kitchen. Marybeth grabbed a deck of cards and dealt a hand of spades. It helped to pass the time, which seemed to be standing still. I felt so helpless. I felt so guilty not being there with him.

I almost jumped out of my skin when the phone rang. Danielle came out of her room before I even had a chance to say hello.

"Hello?" my heart was beating a mile a minute.

"Hi, any word yet?" It was Linda Grant.

"No...I thought that was who would be on the phone now." My voice must have dropped.

"I'm sorry Lau," she said. "I didn't mean to scare you."

I told her that I really wasn't sure on what time they started so I really didn't know when it would be over. It was already eight-thirty so it couldn't be that much longer.

I turned to Danielle. "It's Linda. I'll let you know when they call about Steve." Danielle put her head down and went back to her room. She was just as anxious as I was.

I told Linda she would be one of the first people I called when it was over and got off of the phone.

"I'm not going to make it," I told Marybeth.

"Yes you will," she said. I went to check on Danielle to be sure she was okay. When I went back in to Marybeth, she handed me that cards. "Deal!" she said as she laughed and we went back to playing spades.

About half an hour later the phone rang again, this time it was Dr. Schumaker. "Mrs. Merrow?" he asked.

"Yes Dr. Schumaker, is it over?"

"Sure is, he's in recovery for about an hour and then they will take him up to his room. The operation went well and if everything goes along well, he should be able to come home be the end of the weekend, early part of next week at the latest."

He told me to take it easy and I hung up the phone. I repeated everything to Marybeth and went in to talk to Danielle. Then I made the rounds on the phone with Marybeth glaring at me the whole time. His mother, my parents, his sisters and then Linda Grant. They could tell anybody else that was waiting to hear. Marybeth was right. It did a number on me. Especially when I was asked questions that I couldn't answer, like could this happen again.

Marybeth made me a cup of tea. I was starting to sip it when the phone rang again. Who did I miss? I picked up the receiver, "Hello?"

"Ya Hi!" I couldn't believe it, it was Steve.

He was really groggy and drugged up, but he said that he wanted to call and let me know that he was okay. He knew I would be nervous and thought that if he called I would feel better.

He was right. Just being able to hear his voice made me relax just a little bit more.

He was okay.

FRIDAY SEPTEMBER 18, 1992

Marybeth came again to watch the kids so that I could go to the hospital for the weekend. Hopefully, when I came back, I would have Steve with me. Talking to him on the phone it seemed as though he was doing fine. The doctors had told us that it would be a short recovery this time and that he would be able to go home shortly afterward.

They really hadn't given Steve any real food since the surgery. They were starting him off with clear liquids. Once he was eating, they would be able to judge when he could leave.

Wrong thing to tell him.

SATURDAY SEPTEMBER 19, 1992

Saturday started out miserably and went downhill every step of
the way.

I started out to the hospital early, about nine-thirty. As I
was driving down Storrow Drive it was reduced down to one
lane of traffic. It was bumper to bumper and moving at about
two miles an hour. Just as I was about to hit the tunnel, the
car bucked and sputtered. I put one foot on the brake and the
other on the gas. I caught it before it stalled. It only lasted for
about ten feet. The damn thing stalled out on me.

I threw my hazard lights on. My hands were shaking. All
the cars behind me started blowing their horns. I put the car
in park and tried to restart it. Nothing. I started to panic. Up
ahead I saw a state trooper directing traffic into the tunnel. I
tried waving to him but he didn't see me. I tried the key again.
Nothing.

Cars were pulling out from behind me and passing me on
either side. What else could go wrong? I tried one more time.
I was getting ready to put the thing in neutral and let it roll
behind the barricade to the trooper who didn't seem to notice
I was in trouble. I floored the gas and turned the key. It started
with a roar. I could smell gasoline. I must have flooded the
engine. I didn't care at that point, it was running.

I drove with both feet the rest of the way, leaving my
hazard lights on just in case. As I was pulling into my parking
spot it stalled again. I just let it roll. I didn't care anymore.

By the time I got to Steve's room, I was close to tears. I
told him that if worse came to worse, I would have my Dad

get me home and Marybeth would take him home when they released him.

He was given a food tray at lunch time. A turkey sandwich and some chips. He tried to eat as much as he could but only got through half of it. He said where it was the first thing he had been given that he wasn't going to push it.

He tried moving around a little bit more that afternoon. He didn't want to lose all of the strength he had worked so hard at to build up the last time. We walked down to the lounge a couple of times. It wore him out even though he wouldn't admit to it.

At suppertime he was brought another tray. This time it was spaghetti. He could only get down a couple of bites.

He was starting to make me nervous. He complained of a stomachache. I thought it was due to the fact that he hadn't had anything to eat.

The patient next to Steve had company. His wife was there with their two little ones. I drew the curtain partway in the hopes that Steve could rest and maybe they would be quiet.

A little while later Steve started to gasp for breath and hold his stomach. He was having a lot of trouble breathing.

"What's wrong!?" I grabbed his intercom and buzzed for the nurse. When they answered the page I yelled for them to get in there fast. It seemed like an eternity.

His nurse, Lisa, showed up about three minutes later.

"What's wrong Steve?" she checked his pulse and blood pressure.

"He is having a lot of trouble breathing! What's wrong with him?" I was almost yelling at her.

"I don't know," she replied, "I'll put a call into his doctor." She quickly left the room to make the call. She was back in a moment later with an oxygen mask.

"I've put the call in, we have to wait for him to answer the page."

A moment later another nurse came in to help her. Steve was really gasping for air by now. I was terrified.

The two of them were mumbling to each other. I hated

that. I wanted to know what the hell was going on. "Where is his doctor?" This time I was yelling.

"Mrs. Merrow, calm down..." She was interrupted by someone paging her to the nurse's station. I followed her because I knew that it was the doctor on the phone.

I could only hear bits and pieces of one half of the conversation. I was really starting to panic.

"The doctor on call is in the emergency room and will be up in a few minutes," she said. She looked at the other nurses there and I could tell by the look on her face that she was upset with whatever the doctor had told her.

"Hey, my husband is in there and he can't breathe!" I thought of doing the one thing I knew would get their attention, I grabbed for the phone as I said "Where's Doctor Ogilvy?"

A nurse grabbed the phone out of my hand. "Don't call him. Lisa said there was a doctor on his way up. Calm down, Mrs. Merrow."

"I will not calm down. If there is not a doctor at his bedside within five minutes, I am going to a payphone and calling Doctor Ogilvy that way." On that note I turned and ran back into Steve's room.

There were three nurses with him and someone from the respiratory department. He was getting worse. He was almost blue in the face. I took his hand and told him to hold on.

He squeezed it with all his might. He was in so much pain and he had a look of pure terror in his eyes. I tried talking to him, but the words weren't coming out. He was grabbing at his stomach with one hand and squeezing my hand with the other.

I looked up at the nurse, "Where the hell is that doctor?"

"I'm right here." A woman came around the curtain and sat on the other side of the bed. "Okay Steve let's see what's going on with you." She took out her stethoscope and listened to his lungs.

"It sounds as if his left lung may have collapsed." She looked at the nurse. "Get X-ray up here stat and get a picture of his chest." The nurse flew out of the room.

Steve looked at the doctor, "I've...been trying...to tell

them...it's my...stomach..." He pointed to where he had been holding himself. "It feels as...though it's...something...is pushing...Like it...is going...to explode!" Each word was an effort for him to get out.

The doctor listened with her stethoscope to his stomach. "Okay," she said, "we'll see what we can do to get you comfortable."

She left his room and at that moment X-ray showed up. I was told to leave for a moment so I waited by the door. At that point I had turned to the wife of the patient next to Steve. Her four year old daughter was sitting and watching all of this and I told her that she should get them down to the lounge. She agreed and they left the room.

The x-ray people finished up and I went back to Steve. I took his hand as the doctor came in. I was focused on Steve and really wasn't listening to her. She was going on about how she was going to relieve the pressure in his stomach. I heard her say something about a tube.

I turned to watch her and that's when alarms started going off in my head. She was bringing a tube towards Steve's nose. She said something about it traveling down to his stomach and draining whatever was in there.

I grabbed her hand, "What are you doing? He cannot have anything passed through his nose! It should be in his chart."

Her hand backed away that held the tubing. She looked at me puzzled. I tried to explain. "The type of surgery he had last spring involved his sinuses. Dr. Joseph from Mass. Eye and Ear told us that he could not have anybody put ANYTHING through his nose except either himself or Dr. Ogilvy."

"Okay, I wasn't aware of that." She looked at Steve. "That will mean that you have to swallow this. Do you think you can do that?"

He nodded. I was afraid at this point that he was going to lose consciousness. She told him that she would lubricate it to make it easy on him.

It took him a couple of tries through which he vomited, but he managed to swallow the tubing. When she was done, it drained everything out and he started to relax a little. The entire time this was going on, Steve held tightly to my hand. The more that drained from his stomach, the looser his grip got.

The doctor explained that what had happened was that Steve developed an acute illias. Very common in patients who have been restricted to bed after surgery, she told us. It would correct itself in a few days.

She ordered him a mild sedative to help him relax and hopefully enable him to fall to sleep. Then she was on her way.

A nurse came in to clean Steve and give him some fresh bedding. Steve wouldn't let go of my hand. He was so terrified. I couldn't imagine the fear he had felt. I could only stay with him, hold his hand and pray that it was over. At least for tonight.

I helped his nurse and then stayed until he had calmed down enough to let the sedative take effect. I told the nurse how to reach me if anything happened during the night. I gave Steve a kiss goodnight and headed for my car, silently praying that it was going to start and get me to my parent' house.

It took a couple of tries, but it finally kicked in. I managed to get as far as my parents house before it stalled again. All I could think was that the good Lord must have taken pity on me. What else could possibly happen tonight?

SUNDAY SEPTEMBER 20, 1992

The doctors told us that as far as the surgery itself was concerned, everything was looking good. If that was the only determining factor in releasing Steve, he would be able to go home any day. They were now concerned with the illias as well. Bottom line was that if he could eat solid food and hold it down for twenty four hours, then they would consider releasing him.

Steve was bound and determined to go home. He was fed clear liquids like Jell-O, broth and Italian ices most of the day. He took it easy but managed to hold almost all of what they gave him. He looked so weak and fragile. However weak he seemed to me didn't matter to him though. He insisted on getting out of bed and walking down to the lounge.

He told me that he was going to go home in a couple of days. I didn't know what to say to him. I could only imagine how he felt. He must be so fed up with doctors and hospitals. I could only hope that they, the doctors, wouldn't send him home unless they knew that what happened last night would not happen to him at home.

"How's the car?" Steve asked me.

"My dad took me in this morning," I started to explain. "The thing is on its last legs. He took me to his mechanic to have him figure out what could be done to fix it. It's all in the computer. He told me it wasn't worth it to have it fixed. He feels that it should get us home though. So Daddy will take me back and forth until they sign you out of here."

I had called Linda Grant the night before and told her what was going on with Steve and that my car was about to die. She knew that it was only going to be for a few days more so her and her husband agreed to relieve Marybeth and take care of the kids at the house until we got back. Once again, another good friend to the rescue.

MONDAY SEPTEMBER 21, 1992

For the next twenty four hours Steve set out to impress the medical staff of Ellison Twelve. He ordered solid foods for himself and forced himself to eat about half of each meal. We took a couple of walks down to the lounge. Once we even went as far as the barber shop on the first floor to get his hair evened out.

TUESDAY SEPTEMBER 22, 1992

By Tuesday morning the doctors felt as if he would be able to go home. I couldn't believe it. This man had only been eating small portions for one day. He was pale and weak. He would get shaky and dizzy walking down to the lounge. Steve didn't care, though. He wanted out of the hospital. He wanted to go home and recover the rest of the way in his own bed with his children by his side.

I couldn't fight with him. All I could do was pray that he would be okay. I called Linda and told her we were coming home. I took the phone number of where her husband worked in the event that the car died on the way.

I packed up his things and looked at Steve. "Are you sure that you're okay? Don't screw around. You're sure?"

"I'm fine. Let's go." He buzzed the nurse. She came in with a wheelchair and walked us down to the front door.

It was a quiet ride home. I was scared the car would die. I stayed on the inside lane most of the time. I would keep looking at him. I knew. I knew that he should have stayed for a couple of more days. He was not ready to be doing this.

"How are you doing?" I asked him.

"Okay, I guess. I just feel really tired. When we get back, I think I'll sneak in and go to bed for a while. I'll see the kids later on, okay?"

"Make yourself comfortable in that bed. I don't think I'll let you out of it for a while." I just wanted him to rest and get stronger.

He looked at me. "You know don't you? You know that I basically just escaped from there."

I took his hand. "Yes, I know that. You better not be lying to me though. You better be okay. I'll tell you something else; you better let me know if we have to go back. But yes, sweetheart, I know."

Steve spent the next few days in bed most of the time. He managed to eat three light meals a day and hold them down. I was constantly on edge. Constantly watching him to be sure he was alright.

I prepared my song for the christening of his new God-child, Colleen, on Sunday. I promised his sister that I would be at the church. I wasn't sure if Steve would make it though. He was still a little shaky. She understood. It was more important to everyone that he recovers.

Sunday morning came though, and Steve insisted on going. He had missed so many important things already, Dawn's birthday, her first day of school and the birth of his new God-child. He wanted to be there. Just the church though, not the celebration afterwards. We would go home after the church.

There was one more thing too. Today was our anniversary. Five years married.

As we walked into the church it took a moment for his sister Linda to move. Then she slowly walked to her brother. She put her arms around him and with tears running down her cheeks whispered two words..."Thank you." Whether she was thanking Steve for being there or thanking God for letting him be there, I don't know. It was two words that I had said a lot. Thank You. Thank You, God.

As I stood at the front of the church and sang the song that Colleen's mother had written for her christening, it took all that I had not to break down in tears myself. It was heart wrenching when I saw Steve walking down the aisle of the church holding his God-child with his sisters on either side of him, followed by Linda's husband Tom. Here was this man who had fought to stay alive holding a new life. New hope. It was a beautiful sight.

Thank You. Thank You, God.

Does this end the story? No...not by a long shot. Steve will probably relive a portion of his nightmare every day for the rest of his life, as will I.

Steve attempted to go back to work only to have a coughing fit make his eyes go haywire. He is diagnosed with diplopia, double vision. Nobody really gives him a clear cut answer to it other than that a nerve must have been nicked during the original surgery. Steve accepts it over time, and puts his strength and energy into his children. In his words, he wants to enjoy them while he can. No one can predict tomorrow for him. So he wants to take advantage of all of his todays.

It takes close to two years to fight the legal system and have them agree with the doctors that he is fully disabled. The doctors say that he should watch how much he lifts, not be around dusty, and fume ridden warehouses. They say he cannot deep sea dive, not that he ever had or wanted to, but now we know he can't. Airplanes could be a problem, they are not sure.

A psychologist said that he is agoraphobic. That he cannot be around a large group of people without it bothering him. The mood swings happen now and again, but we survive them.

My thoughts fall back constantly on all of those people who carried me through all of this. How much people gave of themselves. Especially Linda Grant. Right from the start, she not only opened her heart, but opened up her home as well. She gave up two full months of her life to care for my children. I was able to know that while I was with Steve in Boston, my kids were safe. No one could have done more for me than Linda and her family.

Marybeth, who without a thought, would give up her weekends to give Linda a break. Without a complaint, drive the kids down to Boston in my rundown little car so they could see Steve.

Sue, who dropped everything to get me to Steve on that first day. Who stayed with me and was always there when I needed an ear.

Al, making sure that the house was watched. Getting my mail collected and brought to me in Watertown. Transporting me back and forth on the weekends that I went home. Passing the hat and gathering all of Steve's friends together to lessen our financial burden. Most of all finding Rich Chapin, who I will always remember, to donate blood for Steve.

Your mother and your sisters, always there at your bedside helping you to pull through. Helping me out when they could.

The two people that I will never be able to thank enough are my parents. They took me into their home and held my sanity together while fighting to keep their own. They held my hand and listened to my horror stories at the end of each day. They put aside their needs for two months to tend to mine. They opened their door and their hearts again in September. There is no way I could begin to thank them. Nor would they want me to. In their hearts they know that they helped me to survive everyone's worst nightmare.

All of these people and even more, some of whom I don't even know, helped us to survive this and I will never forget that. Every person's prayers and every mass offered in the name of Steve will always be held in a special place in my heart. Even my grandparents, who in their latter years took special time to attend masses and send Steve a spiritual.

Cards, twenty fold, hung in his rooms to brighten his spirit and make him realize all of the special people who were pulling for him. All of the special people who loved him.

No, the story doesn't end here. Hopefully the heartache will end. Hopefully the nightmares will cease at night. Hopefully the fear of tomorrow will go away. As I sit here and complete what started out as a journal, I look to the dresser in my bedroom. On a shelf that is near to Steve's side of the bed. A small purple stuffed dog lies in watch over us. Steve's comforting presence during all of those hellish hours in the hospital...George.

CAN YOU FEEL MY TEARS
A song written by lauri merrow

Can you feel my tears
Running down upon your cheeks?
Can you hear my heart
Breaking into tiny pieces?

Open up your eyes
So you can wipe away these tears.
Take me in your arms
Hold me close to calm my fears.

The last thing that you told me
Was you'd be back before too long.
You bent down to kiss me
"I love you babe" and you were gone.

Then a voice rang through the phone lines,
"Hurry Ma'am he needs you here"
White coats, flashing neon,
Pain and terror filled the air.

They say that you can hear me,
I promise I won't leave your side
Let them pray to save you,
And I'll sing to you 'til morning's nigh.

Days pass on beside us
Taking what they can from you
Don't stop fighting darling
I know our love will see you through.

Dark sky's fill with sunshine
You have now come back to me
You met death at it's doorstep
Slammed the door and took the key.

Can you feel my tears
Running down upon your cheeks?
Can you hear my heart
Breaking into tiny pieces?

We'll hang on to our today's.
We survived the yesterdays.
We'll cherish each tomorrow as it becomes a today.
We still have each other.
I still have my Steve.